Laboratory Urinalysis and Hematology

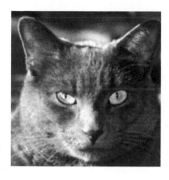

for the Small Animal Practitioner

Carolyn A. Sink
MS, MT (ASCP)
Supervisor, Laboratory Diagnostic Services,
Virginia-Maryland Regional College of
Veterinary Medicine

Bernard F. Feldman
DVM, Ph.D.
Chief, Laboratory Diagnostic Services
Virginia-Maryland Regional College of
Veterinary Medicine

Photographs by:
Donna L. Burton CLA (ASCP)

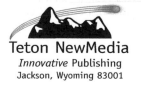

Teton NewMedia
Innovative Publishing
Jackson, Wyoming 83001

Executive Editor: Carroll C. Cann
Development Editor: Susan L. Hunsberger
Editor: Cynthia Roantree
Creative Director: Anita B. Sykes
Production & Layout: 5640 Design, www.fiftysixforty.com
Photographs: Donna L. Burton CLA (ASCP)

Teton NewMedia
P.O. Box 4833
4125 South Hwy 89
Jackson, WY 83001
1-888-770-3165
www.tetonnm.com

PRINTED IN THE UNITED STATES OF AMERICA

ISBN: 9781893441187 (Pack-Book and CD)

Print number 5 4 3 2

Library of Congress Cataloging-in-Publication Data
Sink, Carloyn A.
  p. cm.
  Laboratory urinalysis and hematology, for the small animal practitioner / Carolyn
A. Sink, Bernard F. Feldman.
  Includes bibliographical references.
  ISBN 1-893441-10-5
    1. Veterinary urology--Handbooks, manuals, etc. 2. Veterinary hematology--
Handbooks, manuals, etc. I. Feldman, Bernard F. (Bernard Frank) II. Title.

SF77.S56 2003
636.089'60756--dc21

2003040247

Dedication

This text is dedicated to veterinary students, clinical laboratory professional colleagues, clinical veterinarians, veterinarians who use our services on a daily basis, and all those trained or in training who recognize the immense and needed resource of the veterinary clinical laboratory.

We also dedicate this text to our families.

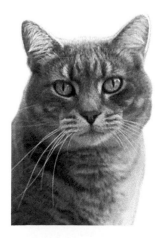

Supplementary Resources Disclaimer

Additional resources were previously made available for this title on CD. However, as CD has become a less accessible format, all resources have been moved to a more convenient online download option.

You can find these resources available here: http://resourcecentre.routledge.com/ books/9781893441187

Please note: Where this title mentions the associated disc, please use the downloadable resources instead.

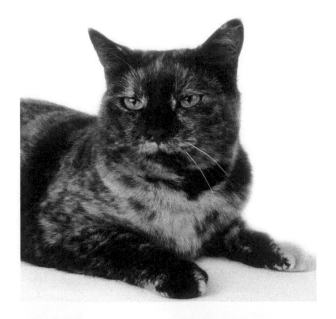

Acknowledgment

Recognizing that no technical book is completely the original work of the authors, we would like to express our appreciation to everyone who gave us direction and helped us understand what would be most clinically useful on a day to day basis. To a large extent, our veterinary student trainees asked so many of the "right" questions. We would also like to acknowledge the atmosphere in our laboratory which fostered this work. Special thanks to Peggy Brown, Laura Fidgen, Janice Herzog, and Jonathan Austin.

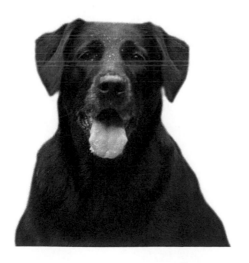

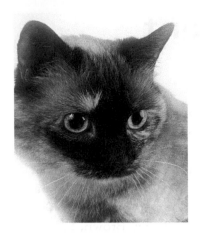

Preface

The veterinary health professional has both the opportunity and obligation to assist patients by understanding what they are experiencing. Keeping this in mind, this text can be used as a reference to help explain routinely used procedures.

In light of developments in knowledge and technical aspects of the veterinary clinical pathology laboratory and the continuing evolution of approaches to veterinary hematology and urinalysis, this material has been created to highlight the fundamental principles of these important aspects of the clinical laboratory. We have included fuller definitions of some critical requirements for accuracy and service to the needs of our patients.

Carolyn Sink
Bernard Feldman

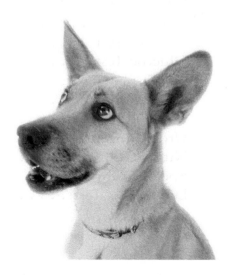

Table of Contents

Urinalysis

Section 1 Specimen Collection and Dipstick Analysis

Section 2 Microscopic Analysis

Hematology

Section 3 Specimen Collection and Testing

Section 4 White Blood Cells

Section 5 Red Blood Cells

Section 6 Platelets

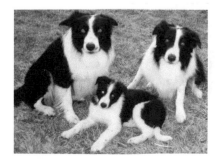

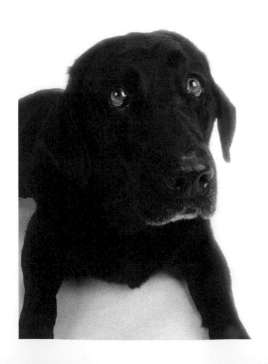

Urinalysis

Section 1

Specimen Collection and Dipstick Analysis

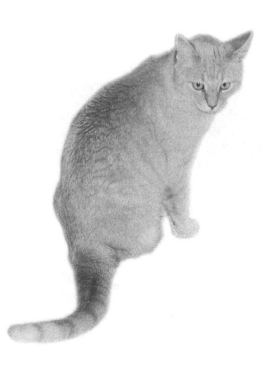

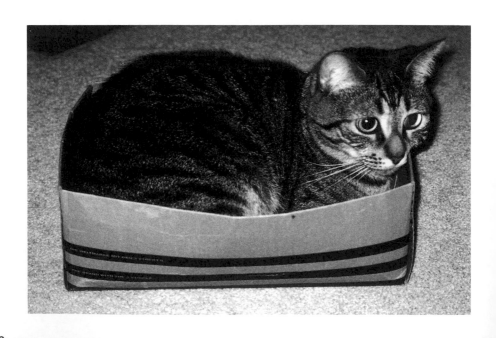

Introduction

The main goal of this book is to provide an easily readable and accessible reference text which we hope will be readily found on the laboratory bench and will be constantly open and used.

Some Helpful Hints

Scattered throughout this text are the following symbols to help you focus on what is really important.

✓ This is a routine feature of the subject being discussed. We've tried to narrow them down.

♥ This is an important feature. You should remember this.

💣※ Something serious will happen if you do not remember this.

⊙ A CD is available as an accompaniment to this printed volume. The CD-ROM allows you to search and retrieve the full text, figures, and tables of the book plus additional illustrations. To purchase this CD-ROM, please call 877-306-9793.

Specimen Procurement

Collection Methods

✔ Urine specimens may be obtained by **catheterization, cystocentesis,** or by collecting **voided** urine.

   ✔ A **catheterized** urine sample is collected by insertion of a catheter into the bladder via the urethra. Urine may be collected through a syringe attached to the catheter or by allowing urine to flow into an appropriate receptacle.

   ✔ **Cystocentesis** may be used to obtain a urine sample. This is performed by inserting a needle into the bladder and aspirating urine via syringe. This method is ideal to avoid contamination associated with catheterization or voided urine.

   ✔ **Voided** urine specimens may be collected as the animal urinates. These are least ideal.

💣 Optimally, at least 10 milliliters of urine should be collected.

Detailed procedures for these methods of urine collection may be found in many veterinary textbooks.

Specimen Containers

✔ Urine specimens should be collected in clean, leak-proof containers.

✔ The container should be labeled with appropriate patient identification information, time, and date of urine collection.

♥ The urine specimen may be collected in one container and transferred to another container prior to laboratory testing. The container used during laboratory analysis should be transparent so that the physical properties of the urine specimen may be easily assessed.

✔ The container should fit into the appropriate centrifuge and possess the ability to be capped in order to prevent aerosol formation during centrifugation.

✔ The container capacity should be at least 10 milliliters of urine.

✔ For routine urinalysis, **do not add** preservatives to the urine specimen.

Specimen Processing

✓ Optimally, laboratory analysis should be performed immediately upon urine collection.

✓ In the event that laboratory analysis is delayed for longer than 30 minutes from the time of collection, the urine sample may be refrigerated at 2-8° degrees centigrade for up to 4 hours.

✓ While refrigeration is routinely used to prevent bacterial proliferation in urine specimens, it may also cause an increase in specific gravity and precipitation of amorphous crystals.

♥ Refrigerated urine specimens should be allowed to warm to room temperature prior to testing. This may dissolve some of the amorphous crystals.

Definition of Urinalysis

✓ Urinalysis is composed of laboratory tests that evaluate the physical and chemical properties of a urine specimen. Additionally, urine sediment is evaluated microscopically.

Physical Properties

♣* Physical properties include urine color, transparency, and specific gravity.

Urine Color and Transparency

✓ Urine color and transparency vary from urine sample to sample. In order to achieve consistency in reporting color and transparency, it may be beneficial to create a list of standardized colors and transparencies so that each member of the technical staff reports the color and transparency using similar terms. Standardizing a "pick list" may eliminate variation. Reporting guidelines for color and transparency are listed below (Figures 1-1 and 1-2).

Figure 1-1 Urine colors.

Colorless

Pale yellow, light yellow, or straw

Yellow

Dark yellow

Amber

Pink

Red

Brown

Dark Brown

Brown-Black

Yellow-Green

Pink-Yellow

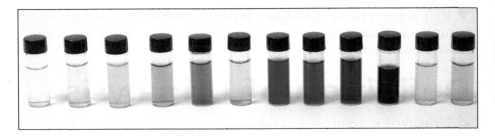

Figure 1-2 Urine transparency.

Clear

Slightly hazy

Slightly turbid

Cloudy

Hazy

Turbid

Flocculent

Bloody

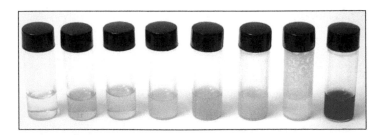

Specific Gravity

✓ Urine specific gravity may be performed by reagent strip method, urinometer, or refractometer.

✓ Reagent strip methodology utilizes ionic concentration indicators and thereby determines specific gravity colorimetrically. Reagent strip methods consume one drop of urine for testing. Specific gravity measurements ranging from 1.000 to 1.030 may be determined.

✓ Urinometers determine specific gravity by comparing the weight of urine to an equal volume of water. The urinometer is calibrated for 20° C and should be corrected for laboratory room temperature variations. Urinometers detect a wide range of specific gravities, but a minimum of 10 milliliters of urine is needed for testing.

♥ Specific gravity readings obtained by the refractometric method measure the density of urine relative to the density of water. This method is widely used as it is a rapid and simple method to measure urine specific gravity. The refractometer is the instrument used to determine specific gravity readings between 1.000 to 1.060. Two to three drops of urine specimen are needed for refractometry testing.

Chemical Properties

✓ The chemical analysis performed as a part of a urinalysis utilizes the principle of dry reagent chemistry.

✓ Dry reagent strips, or "dip sticks," are plastic testing strips with 6-10 small paper pads adhered to the plastic.

✓ Chemicals are impregnated on each test pad; each test pad is chemically different. Each test pad is also impregnated with a visible color indicator.

✓ Testing is performed by dipping the plastic strip into a urine specimen (hence, the name "dip stick;") and the chemical reactions are observed by the color change at timed intervals.

✓ Color charts are provided by the manufacturer of the test strip for interpretation of these reactions.

💣 Manufacturer's directions regarding timed intervals and color analysis must be followed explicitly.

✔ Dry reagent strips are available in a variety of test configurations. Tests include pH, protein, ketones, glucose, bilirubin, specific gravity, blood, urobilinogen, leukocytes, and nitrites.

💣* In general, dry reagent strips are easy to use and inexpensive, but may not be highly accurate.

Sediment Analysis

The microscopic evaluation of the urine specimen provides information in regard to the formed elements of the urine.

✔ Formed elements are the insoluble materials that have accumulated in the urine: red blood cells, white blood cells, epithelial cells, organisms, crystals, and casts.

✔ In order to obtain urine sediment, a urine specimen is centrifuged (see page 20) and the supernatant removed. The sediment is confined to the bottom of the centrifuged test tube; it can be resuspended by gentle mixing using a disposable pipette.

✔ Well-mixed sediment may then be placed on a glass slide for microscopic evaluation.

✔ Reporting guidelines may be helpful for standardizing urinalysis sediment analysis results.

♥ Quantification may be preferable to qualification, since the difference between "few" and "rare" is left to interpretation.

Procedure for Performing Chemical Analysis Using Dry Reagent Strip Method

To perform chemical analysis using a reagent strip:

✔ Remove one reagent strip from the container.

✔ Immediately recap the container.

💣* Be careful not to touch the test pad area of the reagent strip.

✔ Dip the reagent strip into the well-mixed uncentrifuged urine sample. The reagent strip will become saturated with urine.

✔ Without hesitation, remove the reagent strip from the urine sample using the side of the urine container to blot off excess urine from the reagent strip.

✔ Hold the strip horizontally to prevent mixing of the reaction pads on the reagent strip.

♥ Observe the appropriate reaction time interval for each reaction pad.

✔ Read and record results for each test.

Dry reagent strips may be read using manual or automated methods.

Manual Method

✔ A timer should be started as soon as the reagent strip is removed from the urine sample.

💣※ Read time intervals for each reaction pad will be specified by the manufacturer and should be followed **exactly.**

✔ The manufacturer will also provide a color chart to consult in order to grade reactions and report results.

✔ Reagent strips should be read in a well-lit area, but not in direct sunlight.

✔ Reaction results should be documented.

Automated Method

✔ Automated reagent strip readers are an alternative method to visual analysis of the reagent strip.

✔ The reagent strip is immersed in a urine sample as outlined above and then placed in the automated reader for evaluation.

✔ The chemical reactions are timed accordingly and read by the instrument.

✔ Results may be printed or downloaded to a computer.

✔ The automated strip reader may provide a more consistent method of reading a reagent strip since the graduation of color for each test on the reagent strip may be difficult to visually differentiate.

Storage of Dry Reagent Strips

✔ Dry reagent strips used for urinalysis should be stored in their original container as purchased from the manufacturer.

✔ The strips should be kept in this container until ready for use.

✓ A drying agent is included in this container and will assist in keeping the reagent strips free from moisture. Keep the container tightly sealed.

✓ Strips should be stored away from direct sunlight and extreme temperatures.

💣 *Do not* refrigerate dry reagent strips.

Dry Chemistry Methodologies

Dry chemical methods can test for 10 agents—proteins ketones, glucose, pH, bilirubin, blood, urobilinogen, nitrite, specific gravity, and leukocytes.

Protein Test

Methodology

Protein test methodology is based on the principle of protein error of pH indicators. The reagent strip test pad is buffered to a constant low pH. Proteins carry a charge at physiologic pH. A change in test pad pH causes a change in color, which indicates the presence of protein.

This method measures 15 mg/dL to over 2,000 mg/dL (trace to 4+) of protein. Less than 15 mg/dL is not detected and will appear as negative.

Test Limitations

This test methodology is sensitive to albumin. It is not sensitive to globulins, hemoglobin, Bence Jones protein, and mucoproteins.

Expected Values

Normal urine contains small quantities of protein produced by the epithelial lining of the genitourinary tract and a small amount of albumin. The protein in normal urine is usually not in sufficient quantities to be detected by most test methods. Therefore, normal urine should be negative or contain only trace amounts of protein.

Urine protein determination should always be interpreted in association with the urine specific gravity.

✔ A concentrated urine sample can contain enough protein to be measured as trace to 1+ without being significant.

✔ Conversely, a dilute urine sample containing trace to 1+ protein may be significant when the total amount of protein lost is measured.

False positive reactions have been noted in highly buffered alkaline urine specimens and in urine specimens contaminated with skin cleansers containing quaternary ammonium compounds or chlorhexidine. False positives have also been reported in urine from patients who have fever or who have been infused with polyvinylpyrrolidone (blood substitutes.) A variety of drugs and anesthetics may also produce false positive reactions.

♥ Positive protein readings obtained by using dry reagent strips may be validated by confirmatory testing. When equal parts of centrifuged urine and 5% sulfosalicylic acid are mixed, proteins precipitate. The resulting reaction is graded:

> Negative No turbidity
>
> 1+ Slightly Cloudy
>
> 2+ Cloudy
>
> 3+ Turbid
>
> 4+ Flocculant

Urine samples that contain albumin, globulins, glyco proteins or Bence Jones protein will produce a positive reaction utilizing this method.

False negative reactions occur when proteins other than albumin are present. Acidified urine may also produce false negative reactions.

Ketones Test

Methodology

Ketone analysis is based on the method of Legal. Sodium nitroprusside reacts with urine containing acetoacetic acid to produce a detectable color on the reagent pad.

This method measures 5mg/dL to 160 mg/dL (trace to large) of acetoacetic acid, a ketone. Readings of less than 5mg/dL are detected as negative.

Test Limitations

This method detects acetoacetic acid, but does not detect acetone or ß-hydroxybutyric acid. Of these three ketones, ß-hydroxybutyric acid is produced in the largest quantity. Therefore, measured amount of ketones using this method may under-estimate of the amount of ketones present in the body.

Expected Values

Normal urine is negative for ketones. Ketones are end products of fat metabolism. Although mildly toxic, ketones are used as an energy source when carbohydrates are not available or unable to be utilized.

Evaluation of urine ketones is important in the management of diabetes mellitus patients to detect development of ketoacidosis.

False positive reactions have been documented with urine specimens that are red in color or urine specimens containing sulfhydryl groups. Urine containing bromsulfophthalein (BSP) may also produce a false positive reaction.

False negative reactions may be associated with bacterial cystitis, as the amount of urinary acetoacetic acid may be decreased.

Glucose Test

Methodology

Glucose test methodology is based on a two step enzymatic process. In the presence of glucose, glucose oxidase catalyzes the formation of gluconic acid and hydrogen peroxide. The enzyme peroxidase then catalyzes the reaction of the generated hydrogen peroxide with a chromogen to create a detectable color on the reagent pad.

This method measures 100 mg/dL to greater than 2000 mg/dL (trace to 4+) of glucose. Values less than 100 mg/dL are considered negative.

Test Limitations

This test is specific for glucose. It is not specific for lactose, galactose, or fructose. This test does not detect reducing substances or reduced sugars.

Expected Values

Normal urine is devoid of glucose.

Glucosuria may be found:

✓ When the renal threshold for glucose is exceeded due to concurrent hyperglycemia

✓ When the tubular resorptive capacity has declined

✓ In severe hemorrhagic cystitis

✓ In urethral obstruction in cats

False positive glucose reactions may occur in the presence of strong oxidizing agents (often used for cleaning) which may be present in urine specimen containers.

False negative reactions: The reactivity of the glucose test decreases as specific gravity increases; this may vary with sample temperature. The urine sample needs to be at room temperature, if the urine is cold (from refrigeration) the enzymatic test reaction will not occur. Test strip manufacturers differ in reactivity with ascorbic acid; some test strips will fail to react in the presence of ascorbic acid in the urine sample. Ascorbic acid is present in canine urine normally.

pH Test

Methodology

pH test methodology utilizes two chemical indicators to determine urine pH: methyl red and bromthymol blue. When immersed in a urine sample, these two indicators produce clear, distinguishable colors on the reagent pad that correspond to pH ranging from 5 to 10.

Test Limitations

This test is specific for testing pH.

Expected Values

5.5-7.5 for dogs and cats

Diet is a large determinate of urine pH.

✓ A predominately vegetable diet will create an alkaline urine.

✓ A predominately meat or high protein diet will create an acid urine.

Urine pH is a crude estimation of systemic acid base status; however, it is unreliable in many disease states and should not be used as a single monitor of acid-base status.

Urinary tract infection or contamination of urine with bacteria can alter the pH of urine.

✓ Many bacteria (e.g. *Proteus species, Pseudomonas species*) produce urease, which will create an alkaline environment.

✓ Conversely *E.coli* can produce an acid urine.

False changes in pH may be caused by:

✓ Urine specimens containing bacteria kept at room temperature may cause bacterial proliferation and result in a change of urine pH.

✓ "Run over" may occur on reagent test strips when test areas adjacent to the pH test area leach chemicals or color that may interfere with pH test interpretation.

✓ Release of CO_2 upon specimen storage at room temperature

✓ Contamination with detergents

✓ Treatment of patient with furosemide (Lasix)®

Bilirubin Test

Methodology

Bilirubin test methodology utilizes the chemical reaction of diazotized dichloraniline and bilirubin. The reagent pad is at an acid pH. When bilirubin is present in a urine sample, diazotized dichloraniline will couple with bilirubin to produce color on the reagent pad that corresponds to bilirubin concentration.

Results are reported from negative to 3+ (large.) This method can detect bilirubin in concentrations as low as 0.4 mg/dL (1+ or small.)

Test Limitations

When using dry chemical analysis, time is important for the total reaction to take place on the pad; therefore, the color change on the pad should not be interpreted until the time allocated by the manufacturer of the dipstick has taken place.

Expected Values

Normally, bilirubin is not present in dog and cat urine. However, the canine kidney can degrade hemoglobin to bilirubin and the renal threshold for bilirubin is low in dogs. The magnitude of bilirubinuria should always be interpreted in light of urine specific gravity. Trace to mild reactions for bilirubin are common in dog urine with a specific gravity of ≥ 1.040. This is not true for the cat; highly concentrated urine in cats should still be negative for bilirubin. Bilirubinuria in cats is always pathologic.

Bilirubinuria may precede clinically evident jaundice with certain disorders making its detection an early indicator of disease.

False positive reactions may result from atypical colored urine. Chlorpromazine and phenazopyridine may also cause false positive reactions.

False negative reactions may occur due to the presence of ascorbic acid or nitrite.

Bilirubin is a very unstable compound and will oxidize to biliverdin if exposed to light or held at room temperature. Biliverdin is not measured by commonly used tests. False negative bilirubin reactions may occur if the urine is not tested fresh and protected from light.

Blood Test

Methodology

This methodology is based on the peroxidase-like activity of hemoglobin or myoglobin. A color indicator and peroxide are present on the reagent pad. In the presence of hemoglobin or myoglobin, this color indicator is oxidized by the catalysis of peroxide by the peroxidase activity of hemoglobin or myoglobin, resulting in detectable color on the reagent pad.

This test detects both non-hemolyzed and hemolyzed red cells from negative to large (3+).

Test Limitations

This method detects intact erythrocytes, free hemoglobin, or myoglobin.

Expected Values

Normal urine does not contain significant amounts (readings of trace or higher) of erythrocytes, free hemoglobin, or myoglobin.

False positive reactions may be caused by:

✓ Oxidizing contaminants

✓ Microbial peroxidase present in urinary tract infections

✓ Contamination with estral discharge

False negative reactions may be caused by:

✓ Increased specific gravity

✓ Formalin (used as a preservative)

✓ Presence of nitrates

Urobilinogen Test

Methodology

This methodology couples urobilinogen with para-diethylaminobenzaldehyde or 4-methoxybenzene-diazonium-tetrafluorobrate to form detectable color on the reagent pad.

Urobilinogen in the range of 0.2-8 Ehrlich Units (EU) can be detected.

Test Limitations

This test methodology detects

✓ Urobilinogen

✓ Stercobilinogen

Most investigators agree that tests or urobilinogen in dogs and cats are unreliable.

Expected Values

0.2–1 EU is considered normal.

False positive reactions may be caused by dark colored urine samples.

False negative reactions may be caused by:

✓ Formalin (as a preservative)

✓ The absence of urobilinogen cannot be detected.

Nitrite Test

Methodology

When nitrite is present in a urine sample, para-arsanilic acid that is embedded on the reagent pad forms a diazonium compound. This reacts with another embedded reagent (1,2,3,4 tetrahydrobenzo(h)-quinolin-3-ol) to form detectable color on the reagent pad.

Nitrate is present in the urine and is derived from the diet. This methodology utilizes the fact that nitrate is converted to nitrite by the action of gram negative bacteria if present in the urine. A positive result suggests the presence of 10^5 or more organisms per milliliter.

Test Limitations

This methodology only detects bacteruria caused by organisms that reduce nitrate to nitrite.

Expected Values

Normal urine is nitrite negative.

False positive reactions may occur with dark color urines. Urine samples with a high specific gravity or large amounts of ascorbic acid may have decreased nitrite sensitivity.

False negative reactions may be found in urine samples from patients who lack dietary nitrate or in urine samples that have not been retained in the bladder long enough (4 hours or more) for the reduction of nitrate to nitrite to occur. This test will not detect bacteruria caused by organisms that do not convert nitrate to nitrite.

Specific Gravity Test

Methodology

This method utilizes ionic concentration methodology. When cations are present in a urine sample, protons are released by a complexing agent in the reagent pad. These protons react with the color indicator bromthymol blue to produce visible color on the reagent pad.

Specific gravity between 1.000-1.030 may be determined.

Section 2

Microscopic Analysis

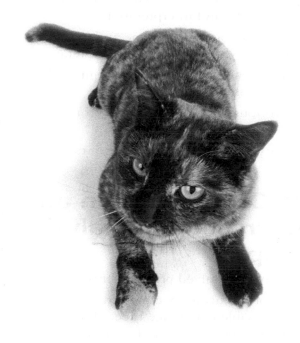

Test Limitations

Reagent strip methodology for specific gravity may differ from refractometer or urinometer readings of urine specific gravity.

Expected values: 1.015-1.040 for dogs
1.015-1.060 for cats

False elevations are found when increased amounts of certain urine analytes are present. Increased ketone concentration or proteinuria of 100-750 mg/dl may produce a modestly increased specific gravity reading.

False decreases may be found in highly buffered alkaline urine specimens when compared to other methodologies for specific gravity.

Leukocytes Test

Methodology

This methodology is based on the fact that granulocytic leukocytes contain esterase. If granulocytic leukocytes are present in a urine sample, leukocytic esterase will catalyze the hydrolysis of an amino acid ester to indoxyl on the reagent pad. This formed indoxyl reacts with a diazonium salt present in the reagent test pad to produce visible color.

Results are qualified from negative to large.

Test Limitations

Trace and other positive readings should be investigated.

Expected Values

Normal urine specimens are negative for leukocytes as detected by this methodology.

False positive results may occur if vaginal contamination of the urine sample occurs.

False negative results may occur if the urine specimen contains cephalexin, cephalothin, tetracyline, gentamicin, or high concentrations of oxalic acid. Elevated albumin levels (>499 mg/dl), elevated glucose concentrations (>=3 g/dl), or high specific gravity of the urine specimen may also produce false negative results.

Centrifugation of Urine Specimen

✓ Urine specimens are centrifuged in order to obtain sediment for microscopic analysis.

✓ The purpose of sediment analysis in a routine urinalysis is to identify formed elements in the urine sample: cells, casts, and crystals.

✓ Consistency of laboratory technique is essential in regard to the procedure used to concentrate the sediment of a urine sample.

For example, variation in centrifugation speed or centrifugation time may affect sediment results and interpretation.

Other technical variables such as storage time and storage temperature may also effect sediment results and interpretation.

✓ When kept at room temperature, cells and casts begin to lyse within 2 hours of urine collection.

✓ When refrigerated, amorphous crystals precipitate from the urine specimen.

💣※ Consistency in laboratory methods is the key to obtaining meaningful results.

Procedure for Centrifugation and Performing Microscopic Analysis of a Urine Sample

1. The urine sample should be well mixed prior to centrifugation.

2. Pour a specified amount of the urine specimen in an appropriately labeled disposable centrifuge tube. This amount should be consistent between samples to assist in interpretation.

3. 💣※ Cap the specimen to prevent formation of aerosols during centrifugation. Balance centrifuge.

4. The urine specimen should be centrifuged at 400G for 5 minutes. Centrifugation time in revolutions per minute (RPM) should be calculated using this formula:

   RPM = (square root (400/28.38R)) X 1000, where
   R = radius of centrifuge rotor in inches

   💣※ Allow the centrifuge to stop slowly. Do not use the centrifuge brake as this may disrupt the sediment.

5. Any necessary confirmatory tests should be performed on the supernatant.

6. If no confirmatory tests are necessary, dispose of supernatant. This should be done by quickly dumping the supernatant in an appropriate waste receptacle. A small amount of supernatant and the urine sediment will remain in the bottom of the centrifuge tube.

7. Using a disposable pipette, gently resuspend the sediment button from the bottom of the tube.

8. Place one drop of this suspension on a glass slide. Cover with 20 mm cover glass.

9. ☀ Allow the sediment to settle for 30-60 seconds before performing microscopic analysis.

10. Perform microscopic analysis at low magnification (10X) with subdued light which is needed to delineate translucent formed elements in the urine sediment. While scanning the slide, continually vary fine focus.

   ♥ This magnification will be most helpful in detecting casts. Scan at least 10 fields of view. Average the number of casts in these fields and report the number and type of casts per low power field (lpf).

11. Move the objective to high power (40X.) At this magnification, all other formed elements of the urine sediment may be observed and identified.

   View at least 10 fields and average the number of elements observed per field. Report the number and type per high power field (hpf).

   ☀ It is important to standardize report terminology and units of measure in order to provide consistent and useful results.

12. Record results.

Elements of Urine Sediment

Urine sediment is best viewed using brightfield microscopy.

Using subdued light for microscopic analysis assists in delineating more translucent formed elements in the urine.

Unstained urine sediment is adequate for microscopic analysis; however, a modified Sternheimer-Malbin stain (SEDI-STAIN®

Becton Dickinson Biosciences) may be used to improve nuclear detail and facilitate differentiation of cells and elements.

The following are descriptions of a variety unstained formed elements that may be found while performing urine sediment analysis.

White Blood Cells

⊙ Any white blood cell that is present in the blood stream may be present a urine sample (Figure 2-1). In routine microscopic analysis of urine sediment, white blood cells are not classified as to type, but knowledge of white blood cellular morphology may assist in identifying white blood cells appropriately.

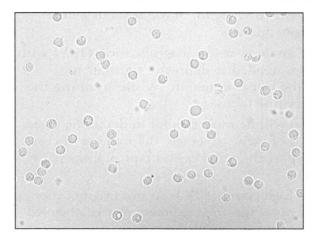

Figure 2-1
White blood cells, dog urine sediment (40 X).

Under high power, white blood cells are circular and are usually 1.5-2 times the size of a red blood cell. The appearance of the nucleus depends on the type of cell present.

✓ Monocytes, lymphocytes, and neutrophils may be present but neutrophils typically predominate.

♥ Nuclear segments of neutrophils may appear as discrete nuclei. The granules of neutrophils may exhibit brownian movement; these are known as glitter cells.

♥ The nucleus of mononuclear cells can be detected as a slight translucency of the center of the cell, unlike the empty center of the red blood cell.

In a freshly voided urine sample, nuclear detail of white blood cells may not be well defined. Microscopic analysis should proceed as soon as possible after specimen collection since cellular degeneration can cause intracellular changes, especially in neutrophils.

💣✳ For example, neutrophils become difficult to distinguish from epithelial cells. By placing a drop of dilute acetic acid with the urine sediment, nuclear detail of the white blood cells may be enhanced to help differentiate them from epithelial cells.

💣✳ With continued degeneration, neutrophilic segments may fuse. In dilute or hypotonic urine, neutrophils swell.

The total number of white blood cells are counted and reported per high power field (hpf).

Red Blood Cells

⊙ Red blood cells are circular and are smaller than white blood cells and epithelial cells (Figure 2-2). Using high power brightfield microscopy, unstained red blood cells in urine sediment appear as pale discs. Red blood cells may be smooth or folded.

Crenation of red cells may occur in hypertonic urine. Alkaline urine contributes to lysis of the red blood cells.

In urine sediment, red blood cells may be confused with fat droplets. However, red blood cells are not as refractile as fat droplets.

Figure 2-2
Red blood cells, dog urine sediment (40 X).

♥ By placing one drop of urine sediment and one drop of dilute acetic acid on a microscope slide, differentiation of red blood cells from fat droplets can be made: red blood cells will lyse with the addition of acetic acid while fat droplets do not.

The total number of red blood cells are counted and reported per hpf.

Fat Droplets

When viewed microscopically, fat droplets appear as refractile spheres (Figure 2-3). Fat droplets are often found in normal dog and cat urine specimens.

Fat droplets are easily confused with red blood cells, but unlike red blood cells, fat droplets typically vary in size ranging from a tiny droplet to slightly larger than a red cell using high power. Fat droplets can be viewed by using the fine focus to vary the plane of view.

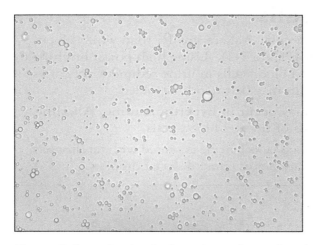

Figure 2-3 Fat droplets in dog urine sediment (40 X).

Fat droplets may be counted and reported using defined qualitative terms-rare, small, moderate, large.

Epithelial Cells

Epithelial cells are large in size relative to other urine sediment constituents.

However the size of the epithelial cell varies depending on its origin. The smallest of the epithelial cells come from the kidneys, ureter, bladder, and proximal urethra.

The largest epithelial cells originate from distal the urethra, vagina, and prepuce.

Epithelial cells may be counted and reported as a group or by type of cells present.

Types of Epithelial Cells

Squamous Epithelial Cells

These are most common in catheterized and voided specimens due to vaginal or urethral contamination (Figure 2-4).

Squamous epithelial cells are large in diameter but are thin in width and tend to fold. The nucleus is small and round; the cytoplasm is large with an irregular outlined cell wall. Squamous epithelial cells may appear singularly or in sheets.

Figure 2-4 Squamous epithelial cells in dog urine sediment (40 X).

Transitional Epithelial Cells

These line the urinary tract from the renal pelvis to the urethra.

The size and shape of transitional epithelial cells vary but they are smaller than squamous epithelial cells and larger than renal epithelial cells (Figure 2-5). The nucleus of the squamous epithelial cell is round and centered within the cell. The cell may appear granular in texture. Occasionally squamous epithelial cells are binucleated. There are various forms of the transitional epithelial cell. They are described by their shape: round, oval, spindle, or caudate. The caudate forms have tails and originate from the renal pelvis. These small transitional cells are 2-4 times the size of a white blood cell.

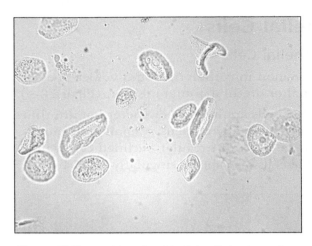

Figure 2-5 Transitional epithelial cells in dog urine sediment (40 X).

Renal Tubular Epithelial Cells

These are cuboidal in the kidney but round once released from the tubular basement membrane.

⊙ Renal tubular epithelial cells are almost perfectly round and are only slightly larger than leukocytes present in the urine sediment (Figure 2-6). The renal tubular epithelial cell contains a single large eccentric nucleus. This cell is very difficult to identify once cellular degeneration occurs.

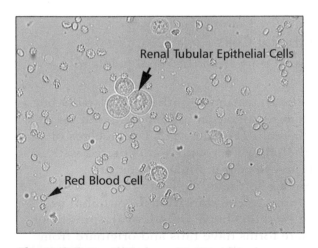

Figure 2-6 Renal tubular epithelial cell in dog urine sediment (40 X).

Neoplastic Transitional Epithelial Cells

These cells are large and round with eccentric or multi-lobulated nuclei (Figure 2-7). They may form clumps or clusters. It is extremely difficult to distinguish neoplastic transitional epithelial cells from reactive epithelial cells (due to inflammation.)

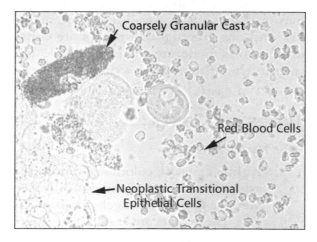

Figure 2-7 Neoplastic transitional epithelial cell in dog urine sediment (40 X).

Casts

Casts are cylindrical shaped. These elements have parallel sides and are the same diameter throughout the length of the cast.

Casts are typically several times longer than they are wide. The ends of the cast are rounded or tapered.

Casts are cylindrical molds formed in renal tubular lumen and are composed of a varying combination of cells and matrix mucoprotein. Cast formation usually occurs in the distal convoluted tubule of the nephron, but casts may also form in the ascending loop of Henle or in the collecting duct.

Casts are named and classified by the cells contained by the matrix mucoprotein of the cast.

There are four criteria necessary for cast formation: acid urine, high salt concentration, reduced tubular flow rate, and the presence of the matrix mucoprotein. Tamm-Horsfall mucoprotein serves as the matrix for most casts present in human urine; this is presumably true for animals. This albuminous mucoprotein is secreted in small amounts by normal tubular epithelial cells in the loop of Henle, distal tubule, and collecting tubule. These are the locations where most casts form. Precipitation of the matrix mucoprotein is the first event in cast formation. Whatever cellular elements present at this location may adhere to the mucoprotein matrix and form a cellular cast.

Generally casts indicate varying degrees of renal changes: renal irritation, renal inflammation, and renal degeneration. Casts may only be seen in a well-darkened microscopic field; two hyaline and one granular cast per lpf are considered normal in a urine that is moderately concentrated. Excessive numbers of casts in the urine implies a disease process in the kidney.

Type(s) of cast(s) per low power field are reported.

Types of Casts

Hyaline Casts

Hyaline casts are colorless, homogeneous, semi-transparent casts with cylindrical and typically rounded ends (Figure 2-8). They are formed from gelatinous mucoprotein and contain no cells. These casts are easily missed microscopically if the microscope light is adjusted too brightly.

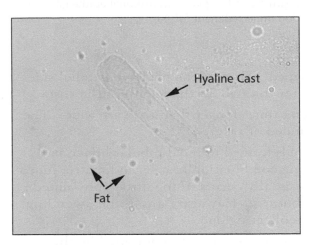

Figure 2-8 Hyaline cast in dog urine sediment (40-X).

Granular Casts

⊙ Granular casts are hyaline casts containing granules which come chiefly from the disintegration of epithelial cells of the tubules (Figure 2-9). The granules start as coarse granules and degenerate to fine granules.

Coarsely granular casts contain larger granules than finely granular casts and are darker in color, often dark brown.

Finely granular casts contain granules that are grayish or pale yellow.

Coarsely granular casts are usually shorter and more irregular in outline than finely granular casts. Coarsely granular casts frequently have irregularly broken ends. It is easy to confuse the coarsely granular cast with clumps of amorphous urates; the cast will have a stronger outline than the clumps of amorphous urates.

Granular casts in the urine sediment usually indicate some underlying tubulointerstitual disorder or proteinuria of glomerular origin.

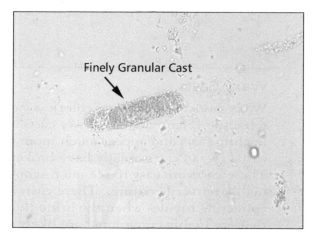

Figure 2-9
Granular cast in dog urine sediment (40 X).

Fatty Casts

Fatty casts (or lipid casts) are a type of coarsely granular cast containing fat droplets (Figure 2-10). These droplets are highly refractile and accumulate in casts as a result of cell lipid degeneration. These casts occur in degenerative tubular disease.

Epithelial Cell Casts

Epithelial cell casts are hyaline casts that contain many renal epithelial cells. They are formed as a result of desquamation of tubular cells that have not disintegrated.

This occurs in any disease producing damage to the tubular epithelium. These casts are sometimes hard to distinguish from white blood cell casts, especially if renal epithelial cells have undergone some degeneration.

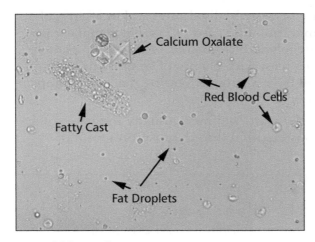

Figure 2-10
Fatty cast in dog urine sediment (40 X).

Waxy Casts

Waxy casts are grayish or colorless casts that are highly refractile (Figure 2-11). Waxy casts are broader than hyaline casts and appear much more solid than hyaline casts. Waxy casts usually have broken off square ends. These casts are easy to see microscopically due to their highly refractile nature. These casts are formed in the collecting tubules when the urine flow is decreased. Casts that are highly convoluted are likely to be waxy casts. Degeneration leading to formation of a waxy cast requires considerable time and intrarenal stasis.

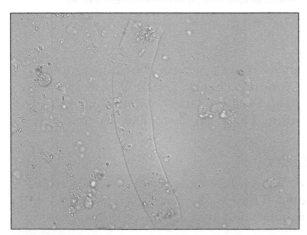

Figure 2-11
Waxy cast in dog urine sediment (40 X).

Red Blood Cell Casts

Red blood cell casts are hyaline casts that contain red blood cells. These casts form when red cells aggregate within the tubular lumen. These casts are rare in dogs and cats and their presence indicates intra-renal bleeding. However, dogs and cats with glomerulonephritis may excrete red cell casts on occasion.

White Blood Cell Casts

White blood cell casts contain white blood cells and their presence indicates a suppurative process in the kidney. Usually, the white blood cells are predominantly neutrophils. These casts can be readily identified unless cellular degeneration has occurred.

Crystals

The presence of crystals in the urine sediment is dependent on many factors: urine pH, urine specific gravity, concentration of the urine with the crystalloid, and the total time lapse between urine collection and analysis. Some crystals are present in urine sediment at room temperature; others precipitate upon refrigeration of the urine sample. Presence of crystals in the urine sediment indicates saturation of the urine with the crystalloid. Crystalluria may be, but is not necessarily indicative of, urolithiasis. Some crystals are only found in certain disease states, but crystalluria is seldom clinically significant.

Identification of urine sediment crystals may be difficult. The first step to identifying crystals found in the urine sediment is to evaluate the urine pH. Normal clinical findings at normal urine pH include uric acid and amorphous urates.

Other normal findings include calcium oxalate found in acid, neutral, or alkaline urine. Hippuric acid may be found in acid, neutral, or slightly alkaline urine; triple phosphate (ammonium, magnesium, phosphate) may be found in slightly acid, neutral, or alkaline urine. Calcium carbonate, amorphous phosphates, and ammonium urates are found at an alkaline pH.

Abnormal clinical findings include: triple phosphate, calcium oxalate, calcium phosphate, urate, cystine and calcium carbonate. Ammonium biurates may be found in alkaline urine specimens and may be present in diseases where hyperammonemia exists. Tyrosine crystalluria is associated with liver disease in the dog; cystine crystalluria is associated with altered protein metabolism.

Sulfonamide crystals may form and are associated with dehydration. Tyrosine, cystine, and sulfonamide crystals are found in acidic urine specimens. Calcium oxalate crystals may be found in acid, neutral, or alkaline urine specimens. The monohydrate form is associated with ethylene glycol toxicity.

The next step in identifying urine sediment crystals involves determining the solubility of the crystal in alkaline or acid. This information is summarized in Table 2-1.

Urine crystals will also have characteristic shapes and may have a characteristic color. This information is summarized below.

Types of Crystals

Amorphous Crystals

⊙ Amorphous urates are found in acid urine. These crystals may appear pink on gross analysis and yellow microscopically (Figure 2-12). These crystals appear as granules in the urine sediment. Amorphous phosphates are found in alkaline urine. These granules are colorless microscopically and also appear granular when viewed microscopically. Occasionally amorphous material may appear in clumps or masses. It may be difficult to distinguish amorphous crystals from bacteria since they may be of the same size when viewed microscopically. However, amorphous crystals are soluble in opposing acid or alkaline solution; bacteria will not. Amorphous urates will also dissolve when heated.

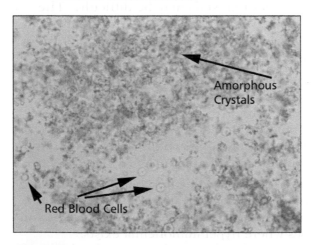

Figure 2-12
Amorphous crystals in dog urine sediment (40 X).

Uric Acid Crystals

Uric acid crystals are found in acid urine. These crystals are yellow or brown when viewed microscopically. These crystals appear as rhombic plates, rosettes, prisms, or are oval with pointed ends.

Calcium Oxalate Crystals

⊙ Calcium oxalate crystals are found in acid, neutral, or alkaline urine. These crystals are colorless when viewed microscopically (Figure 2-13). There are two forms of the calcium oxalate crystal: the monohydrate and dihydrate form. The monohydrate calcium oxalate crystal is described as the "picket fence" form. These crystals are common in ethylene glycol toxicity. The dihydrate form is octahedral or "envelope" shaped.

Hippuric Acid Crystals

Hippuric acid crystals are found in acid, neutral, or slightly alkaline urine. These colorless crystals are prisms, plates, or needle-like in shape. These crystals are often conglomerated into masses.

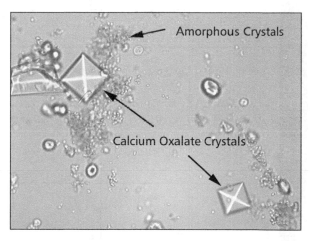

Figure 2-13 Calcium oxalate crystals in dog urine sediment (40 X).

Table 2-1 Urine Crystals: Chemical Confirmation

Crystal Name	Microscopic Appearance	Urine pH	Dissolved By	Not Dissolved By
Amorphous phosphates		Neutral, Alkaline	Acetic acid, HCl	Heat
Amorphous urates		Acid, Neutral	Dilute alkali	
Calcium oxalate		Acid, Neutral, or Alkaline	Hydrochloric acid	Acetic acid
Calcium carbonate		Neutral, Alkaline	Acetic acid produces CO_2 effervescence	
Triple phosphate		Slightly acid, Neutral, or Alkaline	Acetic acid	

Crystal		pH	Solubility	
Ammonium urate		Acid, Neutral	Acetic acid	
Bilirubin		Acid	Acid and Alkali	
Leucine		Acid	Sodium hydroxice	Hydrochloric acid
Tyrosine		Acid	Hydrochloric acid	
Cystine		Acid	Hydrochloric acid	Acetic acid

Calcium Carbonate Crystals

⊙ Calcium carbonate crystals are found in alkaline urine. These colorless crystals are spherical, dumbbell, or oval shaped (Figure 2-14). These crystals appear slightly larger than amorphous phosphates in size. These crystals may be seen in masses.

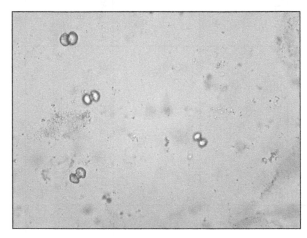

Figure 2-14
Calcium carbonate crystals in dog urine sediment (40 X).

Triple Phosphate Crystals

⊙ Triple phosphate crystals are found in slightly acidic, neutral or alkaline urine. These crystals are colorless and are prisms with oblique ends (Figure 2-15). They are commonly referred to as "coffin lids" due to their similar appearance. Occasionally these crystals are leaf-like or feathery in form.

Ammonium Urate Crystals

Ammonium urate crystals are found in crystals are found acidic or neutral in urine. These crystals are yellow. These crystals are dumbbell in shape or sheaves of needles (Figure 2-16). Occasionally they appear as spheres covered with spicules.

Bilirubin Crystals

⊙ Bilirubin crystals are found in acidic urine. These crystals are yellow, ruby red, or dark brown in color. They appear in rhombic plates, or are needles, plates, or granules (Figure 2-17).

The following crystals are difficult to find without phase microscopy.

Figure 2-15
Triple phosphate crystals in dog urine sediment (40X).

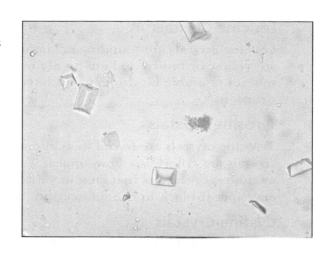

Figure 2-16
Ammonium urate crystals in dog urine sediment (40X).

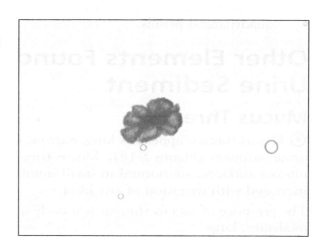

Figure 2-17
Bilirubin crystals in dog urine sediment (40X).

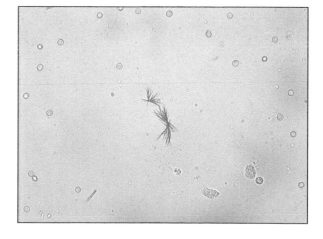

Leucine Crystals

Leucine crystals are founding acidic urine. These crystals are yellow or brown and are highly refractive. These spheres resemble fat droplets but have radial and concentric striations.

Tyrosine Crystals

Tyrosine crystals are found in acidic urine samples. These crystals are colorless. They appear as fine needles grouped in clusters or sheaves that cross at various angles. The clusters may appear black in the midsection.

Cystine Crystals

Cystine crystals are found in acid urine. They are colorless and highly refractive. They appear as hexagonal plates or quadrilateral prisms.

Other Elements Found in Urine Sediment

Mucus Threads

⊙ Mucus threads appear as long, narrow, wavy strands in the urine sediment (Figure 2-18). Mucus threads originate from mucous surfaces, are normal in small numbers, and greatly increased with irritation of any kind.

The presence of mucus threads is usually qualified: rare, small, moderate, large.

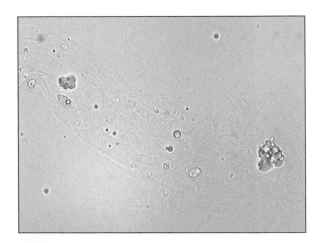

Figure 2-18
Dog urine sediment showing mucus threads (40X).

Spermatozoa

⊙ Spermatozoa are recognized by their characteristic appearance (Figure 2-19).

Presence of sperm in the urine sediment indicates that the urine has been mixed with semen. Sperm may be found in the urine of intact males when collected by cystocentesis.

The presence of spermatozoa is usually qualified: rare, small, moderate, large.

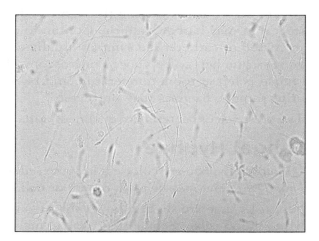

Figure 2-19
Spermatozoa in dog
urine sediment (40X).

Bacteria

⊙ Bacteria are small and very consistent in shape. Bacteria appear as rods or cocci (Figure 2-20). Cocci may chain or cluster; rods may elongate.

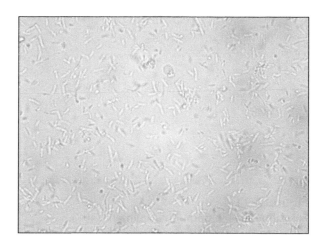

Figure 2-20
Bacteria in dog urine
sediment (40X).

Bacteria may be confused with amorphous crystals; however, amorphous crystals dissolve with the addition of opposing acid or alkaline solution while bacteria will not.

Normally, urine is sterile. Large numbers of bacteria present in a catheterized or cystocentesis urine specimen is indicative of a urinary tract infection. In this case, bacteria are usually accompanied by increased numbers of white blood cells. Bacteruria not accompanied by increased numbers of white blood cells is suggestive of bacterial contamination. Voided urine may become contaminated when passing through the distal urethra or genital tract that may harbor bacteria. Contamination from the urethra in voided or catheterized samples usually does not result in large enough numbers to be viewed microscopically. If the urine sample is left at room temperature and bacteria are present in the urine sample, bacteria may proliferate.

The presence of bacteria are qualified: rare, small, moderate, large.

Fungal Hyphae

⊙ Fungal hyphae are colorless in urine sediment. They appear in varying size and may be oval, round, or budding (Figure 2-21).

Fungal hyphae are slightly larger than bacteria but smaller than white blood cells. Segmented hyphae may be seen.

In general, fungal hyphae are contaminants of the urine sample. Fungal urinary tract infection occurs rarely in dogs and cats.

The presence of hyphae are qualified: rare, small, moderate, large.

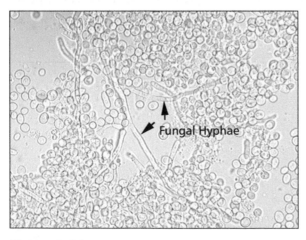

Figure 2-21
Fungal hyphae in dog urine sediment (40X).

Parasites

Parasite ova may be seen in urine sediment. Parasite ova are large elements with distinctive forms.

Possibilities include Dioctophyma renale (kidney worm dog ova), Capillaria plica (bladder worm dog ova), and Dirofilaria immitis microfilaria.

A variety of parasite ova may be seen in the urine sediment if the urine sediment is contaminated with infected feces (Figures 2-22 and 2-23).

The presence of any parasite is noted.

Figure 2-22
Capillaria plica in dog urine sediment (40X).

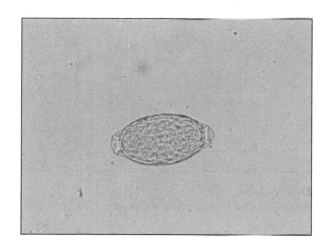

Figure 2-23
Dirofilaria immitis microfilaria in dog urine sediment (40X).

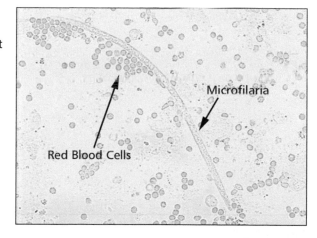

Artifacts

⊙ A wide variety of artifacts may be found in the urine sediment. These artifacts may have acquired during urine collection or during laboratory evaluation. These include cotton fibers, hair, and glove powder (Figures 2-24, 2-25 and 2-26). A wide range of material can make microscopic urine sediment evaluation a challenge.

Typically, the presence of any artifact is not noted.

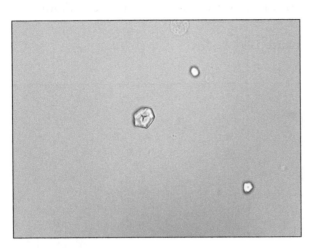

Figure 2-24
Glove powder in dog urine sediment (40X).

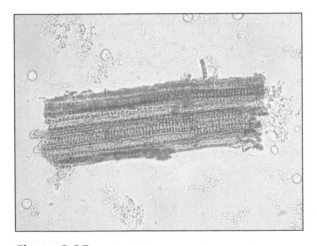

Figure 2-25
Plant material in dog urine sediment (40X).

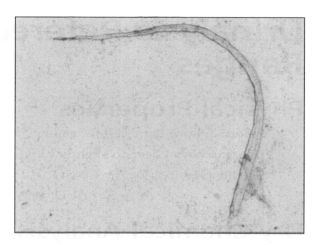

Figure 2-26
Unidentified artifact in dog urine sediment (40X).

Urinalysis Reference Ranges

Physical Properties

Color: Yellow, light yellow, amber

Transparency: Clear to slightly hazy

Specific Gravity: Dogs: 1.015-1.040

Cats: 1.015-1.060

Dry Chemical Analysis

pH: 5.5-7.5

Protein: Dogs may have up to 50 mg/dL urine protein.

Cats: Negative

Blood: Negative

Glucose: Negative

Ketones: Negative

Bilirubin: Dogs may have up to 1+ urine bilirubin.

Cats: Negative

Nitrates: Dry chemistry method is not reliable for dogs and cats; false negative reactions are common.

Leukocytes: Dogs: Method specific for pyuria, but many false negative reactions occur.

Cats: Often produce false positive results

Microscopic Analysis

✓ Results of microscopic urine sediment analysis may vary due to method of urine collection, differences in centrifugation speed, variation in centrifugation time, or urine sample volume.

WBC: Cystocentesis 0-3/high power field (hpf)

Catheterized 0-5/hpf

Voided 0-7/hpf

RBC: Cystocentesis 0-3/hpf

Catheterized 0-5/hpf

Voided 0-7/hpf

Epithelial Cells: 0-3/hpf

Casts: less than 1/hpf

Bacteria: None

Fat: Presence of fat droplets varies; small amount is normal.

Sperm: Present in urine samples taken by cystocentesis of intact males or recently bred females

Mucus: None

Parasites: None

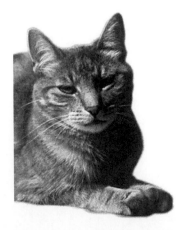

Hematology

Section 3

Specimen Collection and Testing

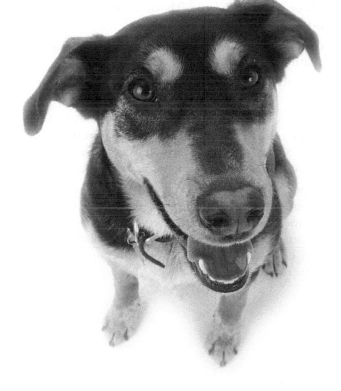

Specimen Procurement

Collection Method

✓ Blood specimens intended for hematologic analysis may obtained through venous phlebotomy.

✓ It is imperative that the blood specimen does not clot. This is accomplished by mixing the blood specimen with an anticoagulant. The anticoagulant of choice for hematologic analysis is etylenediamine tetra-acetic acid (EDTA.)

✓ The blood specimen may be collected directly in to a blood collection tube containing EDTA or drawn by syringe and quickly transferred to an EDTA blood collection tube. The blood collection tube should be tilted so that blood runs down the wall of the tube minimizing hemolysis. The sample should be gently mixed to avoid blood sample coagulation.

✓ The blood collection tube should be allowed to vacuum fill. This insures the correct ratio of anticoagulant to blood is achieved. If the tube is under-filled, excess anticoagulant may create a dilutional effect and inadvertently decrease red cell, white cell, and hematocrit values.

✓ The blood collection tube should be labeled with patient identification information, time, and date of specimen collection.

✓ The blood specimen should be transported to the laboratory for analysis immediately.

✓ When delays in testing occur, whole blood collected in EDTA for cell counts, hematocrit and index calculations may remain at room temperature up to 8 hours. Specimens may be refrigerated at 4° C for up to 24 hours with minimal changes in these values.

💣※ However, blood specimens in EDTA may produce leukocyte changes and morphologic artifacts on blood films if the blood is allowed to stand at room temperature for longer than 3 hours. It is therefore advantageous to prepare peripheral blood smears within 1 hour of blood collection; it is ideal to prepare blood smears immediately after phlebotomy.

Definition of a Complete Blood Count

✓ The complete blood count (CBC) includes all laboratory tests utilized to examine the cells contained in peripheral blood. These tests classify, enumerate, and differentiate the types of cells present in the peripheral blood.

> ✓ Cells are classified as red blood cells, white blood cells, or platelets and counted accordingly. This may be performed using manual or automated methods. When automated methods are employed, red blood cell indicies are usually reported.

> ✓ The white blood cell differential or *diff* is performed by examining a stained blood smear microscopically. Red blood cells and platelets are examined for morphologic characteristics.

✓ Plasma protein and fibrinogen values are often included in complete blood counts in veterinary medicine. This is not the convention in human medicine.

Procedures for Performing Manual Testing

Hematocrit

Hematocrit is the ratio of the volume of the erythrocytes to that of whole blood.

✓ The terms "packed cell volume" (PCV) and "hematocrit" (HCT) are used interchangeably although they are determined differently.

> ✓ The laboratory procedure for determining packed cell volume involves centrifuging whole blood for a specific amount of time in order to obtain red cell packing. The red cell volume and total whole blood volume are measured. This ratio is expressed as a percentage or decimal fraction.

> ✓ The hematocrit is determined by automated instruments.

✓ The packed cell volume may be determined in one of two ways:

Macromethod or Micromethod

✓ The **macromethod** employs a Wintrobe Hematocrit Tube. Well-mixed anticoagulated whole blood is placed in this tube and centrifuged at 2500 G for 30 minutes.

✓ The **micromethod** utilizes a capillary tube centrifuged at 10,000-13,000 G for 5 minutes. The capillary tube is approximately 7 centimeters long and has a uniform bore of approximately 1 mm.

✓ The blood sample used may be whole blood collected directly from a venipuncture or a well-mixed anticoagulated whole blood specimen.

✓ Two types of capillary tubes are available: **heparinized** and **non-heparinized.**

✓ If the blood sample is collected directly from a skin puncture, a **heparinized** capillary tube should be used. These tubes are rimmed with a red line to alert the user that the capillary tube is heparinized. Once the sample is collected in a heparin coated capillary tube; it should be gently rocked back and forth to mix the coated heparin with the whole blood sample. This results in a 1:1000 dilution of heparin.

✓ If the blood sample is used from a heparin or EDTA blood collection tube, the well-mixed sample should be pulled in to a **non-heparinized** or plain capillary tube. These tubes are rimmed in blue to alert the user that a non-anticoagulated capillary tube is being used.

✓ Both types of capillary tubes should be filled and one end should be sealed with modeling clay. Seal-Ease™ and Critoseal™ are two sealing products commercially available.

✓ The filled tube is then placed in one of the radial grooves of a microhematocrit centrifuge head with the sealed end of the hematocrit tube seated away from the center of the centrifuge head. The lid plate of the centrifuge head should be secured and the centrifuge closed and locked. The tube should be centrifuged for 5 minutes at 10,000-13,000G. If the hematocrit is greater than 50%, an additional 5 minutes of centrifugation is needed to ensure plasma trapping is minimized. Once centrifugation has ceased, the capillary tube is placed on a reading device. There are a variety of these devices available commercially, or a millimeter ruler may be used. The total volume of the specimen is measured along with the total volume of the red blood cells.

✔ The **indirect** method of measuring the hematocrit is the product of the mean cell volume (MCV) multiplied by the red blood cell count as determined by automated instruments. This calculation has a greater potential for error in veterinary specimens than the other two hematocrit methods, since in species other than dogs, red cell sizes may be smaller than that of humans and most methods for automated instruments are based on human cell sizes.

Sources of Error

✔ Excessive anticoagulant in blood sample. Excess anticoagulant may over dilute the sample and yield erroneous results.

✔ Failure to obtain a free flowing blood sample from skin puncture. Excess tissue fluid may produce results similar to excess anticoagulant.

✔ Adequate duration and speed of centrifugation. Centrifuges should be calibrated at least annually. Procedures should be standardized and followed by the technical staff.

✔ Failure to mix blood adequately before hematocrit measurement.

✔ Failure to read properly. The red cell volume should be determined. The buffy coat should not be included as a part of the erythrocyte volume.

✔ Irregularity of the inside diameter of the capillary tube. Capillary tubes should be purchased from a reliable vendor.

Macroscopic Examination of the Capillary Tube Using the Micromethod

💣※ When using the microhematocrit method, the blood-filled capillary tube used for hematocrit determination may furnish valuable information in addition to the hematocrit result.

✔ Once the hematocrit result has been obtained, the entire capillary tube may be observed, noting the relative heights of the red cell column, buffy coat, and plasma. The buffy coat is the thin, grayish layer between the red cells and the plasma. This layer includes platelets and leukocytes. A buffy coat of greater than 1% of the total volume in the tube may indicate an increased leukocyte count. While this should not replace an automated leukocyte count, this may be one of the first laboratory determinations of an abnormal leukocyte count. Sometimes a cream colored platelet layer can be observed-often with a magnifier-on top of the buffy coat.

✓ There should be a clear demarcation between the bottom of the buffy coat and the red blood cell pack. If the bottom of the buffy coat is slightly reddened, young cells, reticulocytes, or nucleated red cells are most likely present.

✓ Microfilaria may be detected by microscopic examination of plasma just above the buffy coat. Rarely trypanosomes may be observed at the same site. Observe the intact capillary tube at plasma-buffy coat interface under low microscopic power.

✓ The plasma color should also be observed. Normal plasma is light to dark yellow. Orange or greenish tints may indicate an increased bilirubin concentration. Pink or reddish plasma may indicate hemolysis. Note that poor technique in collecting the blood specimen is the most frequent cause of hemolysis.

✓ Normal plasma is clear; cloudy plasma indicates lipemia.

Hematocrit/Packed Cell Volume Determination by the Microhematocrit Method

Principle

Anticoagulated whole blood is centrifuged to obtain maximum red cell packing. The volume occupied by the red cells is measured and then expressed as a percentage of the whole blood volume.

Equipment/Reagents/Supplies

Well-mixed anticoagulated whole blood

Plain capillary tubes

Seal-Ease™ (Becton Dickinson), Critoseal™ (Kendall Healthcare), or Clay Sealer

Microhematocrit centrifuge

Microhematocrit reader

Procedure

1. Allow the capillary tube to fill with whole blood, at least 3/4 full.
2. Seal one end of the capillary tube with clay sealer.
3. Place the capillary tube in the centrifuge with the sealed end away from the center of the centrifuge head and resting against the peripheral rim.
4. Spin for 5 minutes. A hematocrit value in excess of 50% should be spun an additional 5 minutes.
5. Remove the capillary tube from the centrifuge. A variety of

reading devices are available. Follow the manufacturer's directions explicitly.

6. The total sample volume and the red cell volume are determined. Do not include the buffy coat layer in the red cell volume.

Results

Report results in percentage or decimal fraction. The units are liter/liter, but are frequently omitted from reports.

Plasma Proteins

✓ A variety of proteins are present in the plasma: hormones, enzymes, antibodies, transport proteins, and coagulation factors are just a few.

✓ These proteins possess a variety of chemical configurations and functions, including maintenance of acid-base balance and colloidal osmotic pressure.

✓ Refractometry is commonly used to measure plasma proteins. The principle of this test method is based on the fact that proteins in solution cause a change in refractive index that is proportional to protein concentration.

✓ Refractometers are hand held instruments used to obtain plasma protein values. Most refractometers possess a scale to read plasma proteins directly in grams per deciliter and are accurate in the range of plasma proteins.

♥ Remember that quality control should be performed on the refractometer daily. At least two controls are recommended: one low level and one mid or high level; these are available commercially. Distilled water may be used as a zero point.

♥ Extreme variations in room temperature should be avoided to eliminate erratic readings. Temperature compensated refractometers are ideal.

✓ Plasma from EDTA or heparinized whole blood may be used for plasma protein analysis. Only a drop of plasma is needed. This sample may be obtained by using the residual plasma from the microhematocrit tube used for packed cell volume evaluation.

✓ Clear plasma is required for accurate plasma protein measurements. Since the refractometry method of obtaining plasma proteins is based on transmission of light, any factor that interferes with transmission of light may interfere with a plasma protein reading.

♥ This includes lipemia, hemolysis, and icterus.

♥ Abnormally high concentrations of glucose, urea, sodium, or chloride may falsely increase the plasma protein reading. It is assumed that "normal" concentrations of these analytes will remain somewhat constant between samples and species and be accounted for when reference intervals are established.

✔ Remember that fresh serum contains all the plasma proteins except fibrinogen, Factor V, and Factor VIII, factors which are consumed during clot formation. Therefore serum proteins measured by refractometry will be lower than that of plasma.

✔ Plasma protein determinations that accompany a CBC are helpful in assessing fluid and electrolyte alterations and diagnosing anemia.

✔ Increased plasma protein values are usually increases in the globulin component and are seen in:

Hypovolemia (dehydration)-increase in both albumin and globulin

Inflammation-increase in globulin

Immune mediated diseases-increase in globulin

Some forms of lymphoid neoplasms-increase in globulin

✔ Decreased plasma protein values are usually due to decrease in albumin and are seen in:

Protein losing gastroenteropathy–decrease in both albumin and globulin

Protein losing uropathy–decrease in albumin

Extensive hepatic disease–decrease in albumin

Lack of production of immunoglobulins–often a genetic disease recognized in very young animals.

Chronic hemorrhage-decrease in both albumin and globulin

Plasma Protein Procedure

Principle

Proteins in solution causes a change in the refractive index that is proportional to protein concentration.

Equipment/Reagents/Supplies

Test plasma from spun microhematocrit (PCV) capillary tube or anticoagulated blood tube (EDTA or heparin)

Total solids meter (refractometer)

Distilled water

Lens paper

Procedure

1. Obtain plasma by breaking the microhematocrit tube above the buffy coat or centrifuging anticoagulated whole blood.
2. Place one drop of plasma on the total solids meter plate.
3. Press the plastic cover in order to spread the plasma over the prism.
4. The plasma protein reading is taken from the appropriate graph. (Some refractometers have three scales: one for total protein readings and two for specific gravity readings.)
5. The prism should be cleaned with distilled water and lens paper.

Results

Results are reported in grams/deciliter.

Fibrinogen

Principle

Fibrinogen precipitates from plasma when heated at 56-58° C. When centrifuged, the fibrinogen lies above the buffy coat. Plasma fibrinogens are calculated by subtracting the refractive index of incubated plasma from the refractive index of non-incubated plasma (i.e., plasma protein value).

Equipment/Reagents/Supplies

Spun test microhematocrit (PCV) capillary tube

Test plasma protein value

Total solids meter (refractometer)

56-58° C water bath or heat block

Procedure

1. Place spun hematocrit tube in the 56-58° C water bath for at least 3 minutes. This can be accomplished by placing water in a 12x74 mm test tube and placing the test tube in the water bath or heat block. Be sure that the plasma line of the hematocrit tube is fully immersed in water (but not taking on water.)
2. Remove the hematocrit tube from the water bath after the 3 minute incubation. Spin in the hematocrit centrifuge.
3. Following the plasma protein procedure, read the plasma protein.

Results

Fibrinogen is calculated by subtracting the value of #3 above from the non-incubated plasma protein value. Results are now in gm% (equivalent to grams per deciliter: gm/dL.) Convert the results to mg% (equivalent to milligrams per deciliter: mg/dL) by multiplying by 1000 (moving the decimal point three places to the right.)

Example:

Plasma protein reading   7.4 gm/dL

Reading after incubation   7.0 gm/dL

7.4-7.0 = 0.4 gm/dL

0.4x1000 = 400 mg/dL

Peripheral Blood Smear

✓ Microscopic analysis of the cellular components of blood is accomplished by the preparation and staining of peripheral blood smears. There are **two methods** of preparation: **cover slip** and **glass slide.**

✓ The **cover slip method** employs the use of two number 1 or 1.5 cover glasses (22 mm square) for blood smears.

> ✓ A small drop of blood is placed on one of the cover slips, inverted, and placed crosswise on the other cover glass making the corners form an 8 point star. The blood will diffuse between the two cover glasses rapidly and evenly. Just as the blood has diffused, pull the cover glasses away from each other quickly and firmly along the plane parallel to their surfaces. Cover glasses should be air dried face up.

> ✓ Cover slips may be manipulated for staining by placing the cover slips in a cork. Once stained, the cover slip must be mounted on a glass slide for microscopic analysis.

> ♥ This method of peripheral blood smear preparation provides an excellent distribution of white blood cells with little sampling error.

> 💣 One disadvantage is that the cover slips are difficult to manipulate and require skill and practice to make readable smears. These preparations *cannot* be stained using automated stainers.

✓ The **glass slide method** utilizes two 3x1 inch glass slides.

✓ A small drop of blood is placed on the end of one glass slide. The other slide is used as a spreader. The end of the spreader should be placed in front of the drop of blood and pulled back in to the drop of blood. The drop of blood is allowed to spread toward the edges of the slide and then the upper slide is moved to the opposite end of the lower slide. The smear is allowed to air dry and labeled on the thick end with a pencil.

♥ Remember that some markers are not permanent and will wash off with chemicals used for subsequent staining techniques.

✓ Overall the smears should be free from ridges or other irregularities that would prohibit an even distribution of cells.

✓ There should be a gradual dispersion of cells from thick to thin. Varying the size of the blood drop and angle of the spreader slide will affect the thickness and length of the blood smear. A larger blood drop and larger angle of the spreader slide will increase the thickness and decrease the length of the smear.

✓ An even monolayer of cells is needed for leukocyte differential analysis; a feathered edge should be seen at the end of the slide.

✓ When present, platelet clumps will make the feathered edge look rough.

✓ Microscopically there should be no bunching of leukocytes at the feathered edge.

♥ The benefits of the glass slide method of making peripheral blood smears is that slides are easy to manipulate for manual or automated staining. These smears are also easily read using conventional microscopy.

Peripheral Blood Smear Procedure

Principle

A drop of blood is spread over a glass slide and allowed to air dry. This smear can then be appropriately stained for microscopic evaluation.

Materials

Two clean, dust-free 3x1 inch microscope slides

Anticoagulated blood specimen

Plain capillary tube

Procedure

One glass slide will ultimately be the blood smear, the other will be used as a spreader.

1. Place one glass slide on a flat surface. Using a capillary tube, place a 2-3 mm drop of blood on the glass slide approximately 1 cm from one end.

2. Use the thumb and forefinger to secure this slide on the flat surface. Using the other hand, place one end of the spreader slide just in front of the drop of blood.

3. Hold the spreader slide at 30-45° angle and draw back into the drop of blood.

4. Allow the drop of blood to spread, stopping short of the edges of the slide.

5. Using a precise and evenly weighted motion, move the spreader slide towards the end of the other slide. The entire blood smear should cover approximately 3/4 of the slide.

6. Allow the smear to air dry.

7. Label the thick end of the smear with a pencil.

Discussion

The thickness of the smear is controlled by three variables; angle of the spreader slide, speed of spreading, and size of the drop of blood. In a good blood smear, transition from the thick area is gradual. There should be an even distribution of cells with no areas containing ridges or holes. This is the area of the peripheral blood smear that should be used when performing a WBC differential (Figure 3-2). Figures 3-1 and 3-3 represent areas that should not be used for performing the differential.

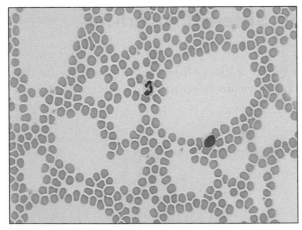

Figure 3-1
Thin peripheral blood smear (modified Wright's stain, 50X).

Figure 3-2
Just right peripheral blood smear (modified Wright's stain, 50X).

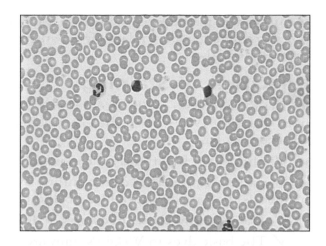

Figure 3-3
Too thick peripheral blood smear (modified Wright's stain, 50X).

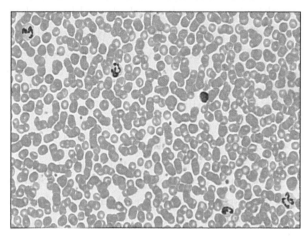

Methods of Staining the Smear

✓ A peripheral blood smear may be stained by **manual** or **automated** methods.

✓ For **manual** methods, manufacturers directions should always be followed, but in general terms, the peripheral blood smear will be fixed, stained, and washed by a process that takes approximately 10 minutes.

> ✓ Stain may precipitate from solution during storage. It may be necessary to filter stain before each use.

> ✓ Stain and staining solutions should be refreshed or replaced as specified by the manufacturer.

> ✓ Coplin jars should be cleaned thoroughly at least as often as the stain is replaced.

✓ **Automated** methods use stainers that provide speed and consistency in staining but are relatively expensive when compared to manual methods.

Principles of Staining

✓ The Romanowski method of staining blood films was popular until the early 1970's when the Giemsa and Wright methods became popular.

✓ Wright's Stain is currently the most common and widely used.

✓ The staining properties of the aniline dyes used in this method is the basis of white blood cell differentiation.

    ✓ There are **two classes of dyes** used: **basic** dyes and **acid** dyes.

    ✓ The basic dyes in Wright's stain are a complex mixture of thiazines, mostly methylene blue and azure B.

    ✓ The acid dye is a methyl alcohol solution of eosin.

    ✓ When nuclei and other structures in peripheral blood smears take up basic dyes, they are named basophilic; structures that take up acidic dyes are termed acidophilic or eosinophilic.

    ✓ Other nuclear structures that are stained by a combination of the two are called neutrophilic.

    ✓ Collectively, these terms are used to classify leukocytes: **basophilic, eosinophilic,** and **neutrophilic.**

✓ Once stained, the peripheral blood smear will appear pink macroscopically.

✓ Microscopically

    RBCs should be pink

    Nuclei of WBCs should be purple-blue

    Neutrophilic granules should be violet-pink

    Eosinophilic granules should be orange-red

    Basophilic granules should be purple

    Platelets should be purple-blue

    Areas with no cells should be clear and there should be no stain precipitate

Troubleshooting Staining Problems

Problem

Excessive pink-nuclei are pale gray or pale blue, RBCs are bright red or orange, eosinophil granules are bright red

Possible Cause

Stain, buffer, or water too acid

Insufficient stain, prolonged washing

Mounting coverslip slides before they are dry

Solution

Check pH of solutions, replace as necessary

Vary stain and wash times, evaluate effect

Vary smear preparation techniques

Problem

Excessively blue-nuclear chromatin blue to black, RBCs blue or green, eosinophil granules are deep gray or blue

Possible Cause

Stain, buffer, or water too alkaline

Prolonged staining, inadequate washing, smears too thick

Solution

Check pH of solutions, replace as necessary

Vary stain and wash times, evaluate effect

Vary smear preparation techniques

Problem

All cells pale

Possible Cause

Understaining

Excessive washing

Solution

Vary stain and wash times, evaluate effect

Problem

Stain precipitate

Possible Cause

Inadequate wash

Solution

Use clean lint-free slides

Vary stain wash times and evaluate effect

Problem

Refractile areas on red blood cells

Possible Cause

Diluted stain (water artifact)

Solution

Use fresh stain regularly, either daily or weekly

Estimating Total White Cell Count and Platelet Count from the Peripheral Blood Smear

✓ A visual **estimate** of the white blood cell count should be performed to confirm automated counts. This estimate may also be performed when automated analysis is not readily available.

✓ Find the portion of the stained peripheral blood smear where the red cells are spread out forming a monolayer of cells. Using the 50X objective, count the average number of leukocytes in each of 10 fields. Using the following formula, estimate the total count: Average number of leukocytes/field X 2000 = number of leukocytes/uL.

✓ Platelets may be estimated in the same way. Use the 100X objective and average the total number of platelets in each of 10 fields. Using the following formula, estimate the total count: Average number of platelets /field X 20000 = number of platelets/uL.

Section 4
White Blood Cells

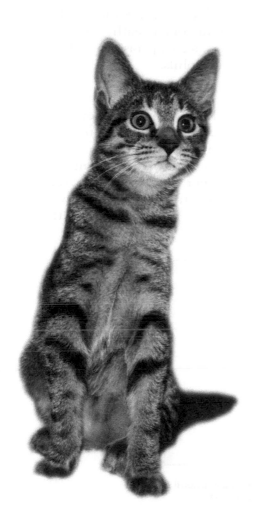

Function and Physical Characteristics

✓ White blood cells are also known as leukocytes.

Neutrophils

Function

Mature neutrophils are released from the bone marrow into the peripheral blood. They transmigrate through the vascular endothelium and serve as the first line defense against microbial invasion. Neutrophils are responsible for both phagocytosis and microbiocidal action which includes chemotaxis followed by ingestion and degranulation, ultimately leading to microbial death. This action is not limited to bacteria as fungi, yeasts, algae, parasites, and viruses may be damaged or destroyed by neutrophils.

Description

Neutrophils are the most common leukocyte in the peripheral blood of dogs and cats (Figures 4-1 and 4-2). Segmented neutrophils are approximately 10-12 μm in diameter. The single nucleus has several indentations that divides the nucleus into lobes. There are typically 3-5 lobes per nucleus. When Wright's stained, the nucleus of the neutrophil stains dark purple with dense chromatin. The cytoplasm stains pinkish-purple with small granules present.

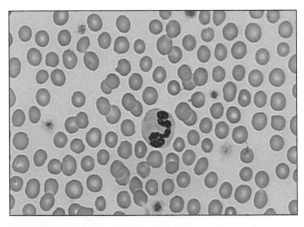

Figure 4-1 Cat segmented neutrophil in peripheral blood smear (modified Wright's stain, 100X).

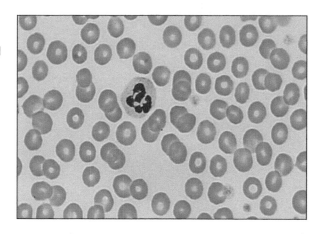

Figure 4-2
Dog segmented neutrophils in peripheral blood smear (modified Wright's stain, 100X).

Lymphocytes

Function

Lymphocytes are the first line immunologic defense of the peripheral blood. There are essentially two types of lymphocytes: T cells and B cells. T cells circulate throughout the blood and lymph systems, while B cells typically reside in secondary lymph tissues (such as lymph nodes.) There is no difference morphologically between T and B cells.

Description

Lymphocytes are smaller in size than neutrophils, but larger than red blood cells. When Wright's stained, lymphocytes have a blue to deep blue cytoplasm, which may possess small pinkish-purple granules. The nucleus is deep purple with dense chromatin (Figures 4-3 and 4-4).

Figure 4-3
Cat lymphocytes in peripheral blood smear (modified Wright's stain, 100X).

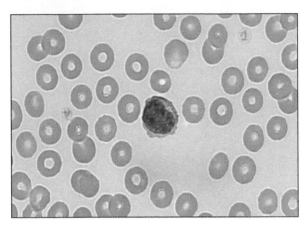

Figure 4-4 Dog lymphocyte in peripheral blood smear (modified Wright's stain, 100X).

Monocytes

Function

Monocytes phagocytize and digest foreign material, cellular debris, and dead cells. In the defense against microbial invasion, monocytes are less efficient phagocytes than neutrophils.

Monocytes are released into the peripheral blood from the bone marrow. Once in circulation, monocytes may leave the peripheral blood in the absence of inflammation, or they may exit circulation in response to inflammation. Once monocytes are distributed to surrounding tissue, they transform to macrophages which contain more proteolytic enzymes and granules than the precursor monocyte. Macrophages are rarely encountered in blood but may be observed in capillary blood smears in disorders such as ehrlichiosis, histoplasmosis, and leishmaniasis.

Description

Monocytes are less common than neutrophils or lymphocytes in the peripheral blood of dogs or cats. Monocytes are between 15-20 µm in diameter in size. When Wright's stained, the large cytoplasm is purple-pink and possesses fine granules described as having a "ground glass" appearance. The nucleus may be oval or "kidney bean" shaped (Figures 4-5 and 4-6).

Figure 4-5
Cat monocyte in peripheral blood smear (modified Wright's stain 100X).

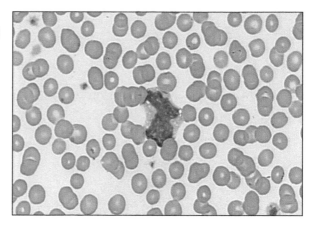

Figure 4-6
Dog monocyte in peripheral blood smear (modified Wright's stain, 100X).

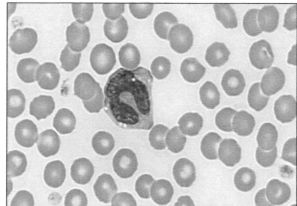

Eosinophils

Function

Eosinophils possess phagocytic and bactericidal properties but are less effective in these processes than neutrophils. Eosinophils attach to and kill helminthes and are attracted by chemical mediators liberated by mast cells during allergic and anaphylactic reactions.

Morphology

⊙ Eosinophils are present in low numbers in normal animals. They are similar in size to neutrophils or slightly larger than neutrophils. Eosinophils are easy to recognize when Wright's stained, as the cytoplasmic granules stain bright red. Cat eosinophil granules may be more ovoid than the dog (Figure 4-7). Dog eosinophil granules are round and quite variable in size and number (Figures 4-8 and 4-9). The nucleus of the eosinophil is similar to the neutrophil in that it is segmented, but the segments may not be well defined.

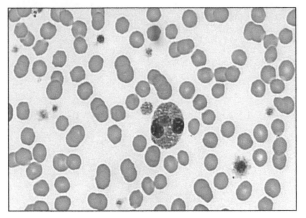

Figure 4-7
Cat eosinophil in peripheral blood smear (modified Wright's stain, 100X).

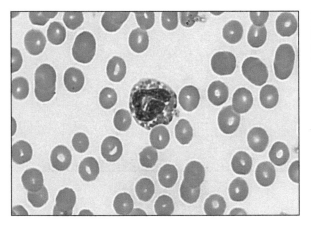

Figure 4-8
Dog eosinophil in peripheral blood smear (modified Wright's stain, 100X).

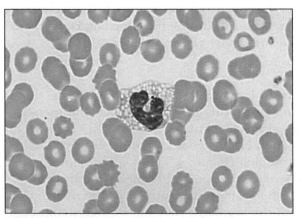

Figure 4-9
Dog eosinophil degranulating in peripheral blood smear (modified Wright's stain, 100X).

Basophils

Function

Basophils are a source of mediators of inflammation. If present, they are present in small numbers in peripheral blood.

Morphology

⊙ Basophils are seldom seen in peripheral blood. They are similar in size to the neutrophil. When Wright's stained, the basophil has a light purple cytoplasm. Few small, round, purple cytoplasmic granules may be present in canine basophils. These are absent in feline basophils. The nucleus is segmented but not to the extent of mature neutrophils (Figures 4-10, 4-11, and 4-12).

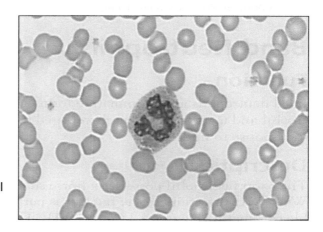

Figure 4-10
Cat basophil in peripheral blood smear (modified Wright's stain, 100X).

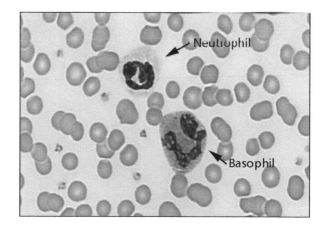

Figure 4-11
Cat segmented neutrophil, and basophil in peripheral blood smear (modified Wright's stain, 100X).

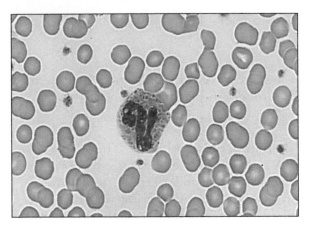

Figure 4-12 Dog basophil in peripheral blood smear (modified Wright's stain, 100X).

Band Neutrophils

Function

Band neutrophils are an immature form of the segmented neutrophil and may be prematurely released from the bone marrow in response to infection.

Description

The band neutrophil possesses a horse shoe shaped nucleus. When Wright's stained, the nucleus is purple and contains visible chromatin (Figures 4-13 and 4-14). The cytoplasm is light pink to purple and may contain small granules which may be difficult to discern.

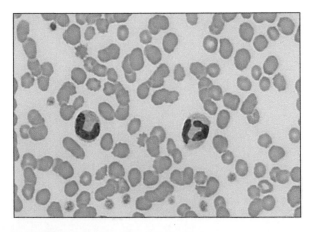

Figure 4-13
Cat band and segmented neutrophil in peripheral blood smear (modified Wright's stain, 100X).

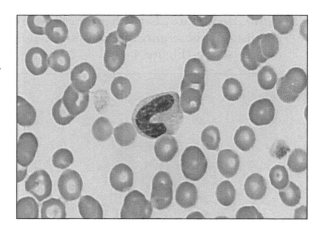

Figure 4-14
Dog band neutrophil in peripheral blood smear (modified Wright's stain, 100X).

White Blood Cell Descriptive Terms

The following terms are used to describe variation in leukocyte morphology.

✓ Toxic change

During the inflammatory process, granulocytes may undergo morphologic changes known as toxic change. These changes include increased basophilia of neutrophilic granules and increased number of vacuoles in the neutrophilic cytoplasm (Figure 4-15).

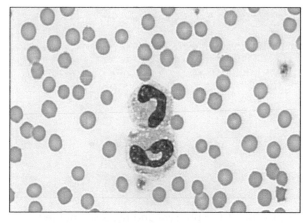

Figure 4-15 Toxic changes in cat peripheral blood smear (modified Wright's stain, 100X).

Döhle Bodies are also indicator of toxic change. Döhle bodies are discrete, blue-gray cytoplasmic inclusions that are round or oval in shape (Figure 4-16).

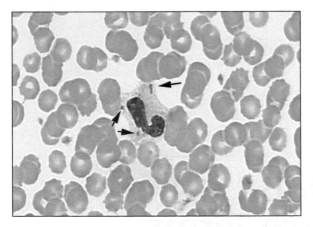

Figure 4-16 Döhle bodies in dog peripheral blood smear (modified Wright's stain, 100X).

✓ Hypersegmented neutrophils

Neutrophils that are hypersegmented contain more than 4 nuclear lobes or segments. Hypersegmented neutrophils are cells which have been in circulation longer than normal (Figure 4-17).

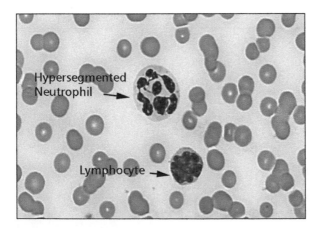

Figure 4-17 Lymphocyte and hypersegmented neutrophil in cat peripheral blood smear (modified Wright's stain, 100X).

✓ Atypical lymphocytes

This term is used to describe lymphocytes that are morphologically different than normal lymphocytes. This includes lymphocytes which are normal in size, but possess an extremely dense nucleus and a deep blue cytoplasm. These cells may also be called reactive lymphocytes or immunocytes (Figure 4-18). Cells with a larger, less dense nucleus with increased cytoplasm may also be called atypical lymphocytes.

✓ Mast cell

Mast cells are easily recognized due to abundant deep purple granules contained in the cytoplasm. The nucleus of the mast cell is often unseen due to the density of the cytoplasmic granules (Figure 4-19).

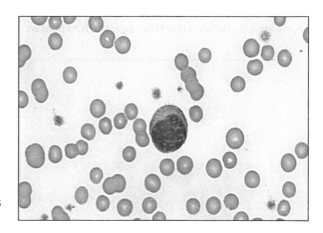

Figure 4-18
Atypical lymphocyte in cat peripheral blood smear (modified Wright's stain, 100X).

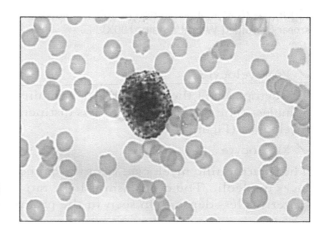

Figure 4-19
Mast cell in cat peripheral blood smear (modified Wright's stain, 100X).

Neutrophil Maturation Sequence

The following maturation sequence is provided for morphologic recognition of immature cells in the neutrophilic cell line. Leukocyte production is beyond the scope of this text and is described in many veterinary hematology textbooks. The reader is encouraged to utilize these references for confirmation of abnormal findings.

Granulocytic Series

✓ Myeloblast

The myeloblast is slightly oval in shape. This cell is composed of blue cytoplasm with a large nucleus which contains prominent nucleoli within fine open chromatin (Figure 4-20).

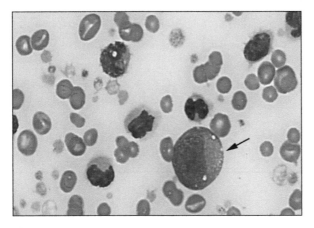

Figure 4-20 Myeloblast in dog peripheral blood smear (modified Wright's stain, 100X).

✓ Promyelocyte

The cytoplasm of the promyelocyte contains both pink and purple granules. The nucleus contains less distinct nucleoli than the myeloblast (Figure 4-21).

✓ Myelocyte

The neutrophilic myelocyte contains an eccentric nucleus which lacks nucleoli. The cytoplasm is light tan color and the granular pattern is less dense than seen in the promyelocyte (Figure 4-22).

Figure 4-21
Promyelocyte in dog peripheral blood smear (modified Wright's stain, 100X).

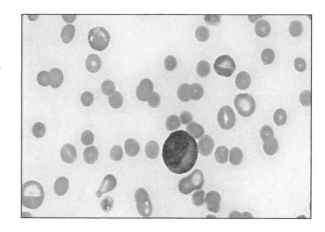

Figure 4-22
Myelocyte in dog peripheral blood stain (modified Wright's stain, 100X).

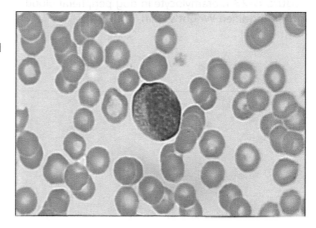

✓ Metamyelocyte

The metamyelocyte contains an indented nucleus with azurophilic cytoplasmic granules (Figure 4-23).

✓ Band neutrophil

The band neutrophil possesses a horse shoe-shaped nucleus. The horse shoe-shaped nucleus is purple and contains visible chromatin. The cytoplasm is light pink to purple and may contain small granules (Figure 4-24).

✓ Segmented neutrophil

The single nucleus of the segmented nucleus has several indentations that divides the nucleus into 3-5 lobes (see Figure 4-24). The nucleus stains dark purple with dense chromatin. The cytoplasm stains pinkish-purple with small granules present.

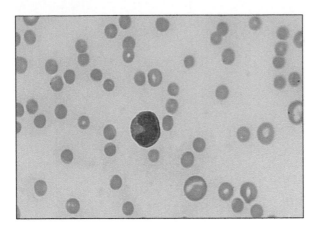

Figure 4-23 Metamylocyte in dog peripheral blood smear (modified Wright's stain, 100X).

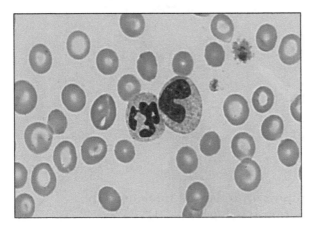

Figure 4-24 Segmented and band neutrophil in dog peripheral blood smear (modified Wright's smear, 100X).

Section 5
Red Blood Cells

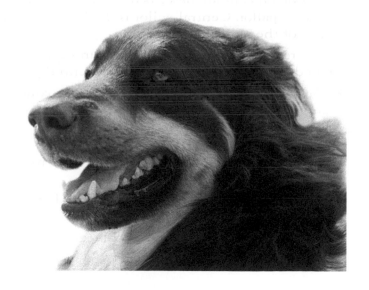

Function and Physical Characteristics

Function

✓ Red blood cells serve as oxygen transport vehicles by acquiring oxygen in the lung, carrying oxygen to oxygen deprived cells throughout the body, exchanging it for carbon dioxide, and carrying carbon dioxide back to the lung for release via expiration.

✓ This cycle is continuous and is repeated for the life of the red blood cell.

✓ Hemoglobin is the main component of red blood cells and is responsible for oxygen and carbon dioxide transportation.

    ✓ Each hemoglobin molecule is composed of:

        Heme-4 groups, each containing 1 atom of ferrous iron. Each heme group is located near the surface of the molecule, and is responsible for reversibly combining with 1 molecule of oxygen or carbon dioxide.

        Globin-2 pairs of polypeptide chains

Physical Characteristics

✓ Red blood cells are anuclear biconcave discs that stain red to reddish orange with Wright's stain.

✓ Red blood cells are described by their size, shape, and degree of central pallor. Central pallor is the lighter staining area in the middle of the red cell.

✓ Dog red blood cells are consistent in size, are approximately 7 μm in diameter, and have prominent central pallor.

✓ Cat red blood cells vary in size, are approximately 5 μm in diameter, and have less central pallor than dogs.

Specimen Collection

✓ Blood specimens should be collected using routine phlebotomy technique.

✓ Whole blood is necessary for obtaining hemoglobin values and red blood cell counts.

✓ EDTA is the anticoagulant of choice.

Laboratory Analysis

✓ Red blood cells may be enumerated by **manual** or **automated** methods.

✓ For the **manual method,** red blood cells are counted microscopically using a hemacytometer.

A well-mixed EDTA anticoagulated blood specimen is diluted 1:200 in 0.85% ammonium oxalate solution.

A hemacytometer is charged.

Red blood cells appear as round cells microscopically.

Red blood cells are counted in 5 small squares of the center square.

The number of red blood cells per cubic millimeter (1 cubic millimeter=1 microliter), is calculated as follows:

Number of cells counted x Dilution (200) x Depth (10) x 5 (1/5 of square mm counted)

Example:

450 red blood cells are counted in the 5 small squares of the center square.

Calculation: Total number of red blood cells = 450 x 200 x 10 x 5

Result: Total number of red blood cells = 4,500,000 Red blood cells per cubic millimeter

The Unopette system (Becton- Dickinson, Rutherford, NJ) is available commercially.

The manual method of red blood cell analysis is tedious and prone to inaccuracy. Due to this fact, many clinical laboratories had eliminated the manual red blood cell count from the CBC before the advent of automated technology.

✓ For the **automated method,** red blood cells are counted by electrical impedance

♥ Coulter developed and first marketed the electrical impedance method in the early 1960s. This method is no longer limited to Coulter instruments and is widely used today.

♥ In automated systems using electrical impedance, anticoagulated whole blood is diluted in an electrolyte solution. The resulting solution of blood cells are routed through a small opening between two electrodes. This opening is known as the aperture. A precise volume of diluted blood is moved through the aperture for a precise time period. As red blood cells are moved across the aperture, they inhibit the flow of electrical current across that aperture. The detected changes in current are counted as red blood cells. These changes are accumulated by the instrument and ultimately reported as the red blood cell count.

✓ Hemoglobin may be assessed using **manual** or **automated** methods.

   ✓ For **manual** methods, hemoglobin is determined colorimetrically.

A modified cyanmethemoglobin method is available commercially (Unopette, Becton- Dickinson, Rutherford, NJ). This is a convenient and stable standard solution.

For this method, whole blood is diluted with the appropriate diluent and read spectrophotometrically (540 nm). The concentration of hemoglobin is determined using a curve derived from known hemoglobin concentrations.

Due to the excessive amount of time involved, this method for determining hemoglobin may not be practical for the clinical laboratory setting.

   ✓ For **automated** hemoglobin methods, the same testing principles apply.

A whole blood specimen is aspirated and mixed with an electrolyte solution. Another reagent is added which lyses the red blood cells. Subsequently, hemoglobin is released. Spectrophotometry is used to measure the concentration of hemoglobin in the solution.

Hematocrit determinations are described in Section 4.

Red Blood Cell Indicies

✓ Most automated instruments calculate and report red blood cell indicies.

♥ Red blood cell indicies are useful in classification of anemias.

✓ By obtaining the patient's red blood cell count, hemoglobin, and hematocrit, red blood cell indicies may be calculated as follows:

Mean Corpuscular Volume (MCV in femtoliters (fL)) =
$$\frac{\text{Hematocrit (in percent) x 10}}{\text{Red Cell Count (in millions)}}$$

Mean Corpuscular Hemoglobin (MCH in picograms (pg)) =
$$\frac{\text{Hemoglobin (in grams per deciliter) x 10}}{\text{Red Cell Count (in millions)}}$$

Mean Corpuscular Hemoglobin Concentration (MCHC in grams per deciliter (g/dL)) =

$$\frac{\text{Hemoglobin (in grams per deciliter) X 100}}{\text{Hematocrit (in per cent)}}$$

Example:

5 year old cat has a red blood cell count of 9.79 million per cubic millimeter, hemoglobin of 15.5 g/dL and hematocrit of 44.2%.

MCV = (44.2 X 10) / 9.79
MCV = 45.1 fl

MCH = (15.5 X 10) / 9.79
MCH = 15.8 pg

MCHC = (15.5 X 100) / 44.2
MCHC = 35.1 g/dL

✓ MCV is the average volume of an individual red blood cell. It is an indicator of cell size. This value, when compared to the species-specific reference interval, allows the red blood cells to be classified as:

♥ Normocytic: value falls within the reference interval, red cells of average size

♥ Microcytic: value is less than the lower limit of the reference interval, red cells smaller than average size

♥ Macrocytic: value is greater than the upper limit of the reference interval, red cells are larger than average size

✓ MCH is the average weight of hemoglobin in an individual red blood cell.

♥ A MCH value that is less than the lower end of the species-specific reference interval indicates that red cells possess less than the average weight of hemoglobin.

♥ A MCH value that is greater than the upper end of the reference interval indicates that red blood cells have more than average weight of hemoglobin.

✓ MCHC is the average concentration of hemoglobin in individual red blood cells. This value, when compared to species-specific reference interval allows red blood cells to be classified as:

♥ Normochromic: value falls within the reference interval, red blood cells are of average hemoglobin concentration

♥ Hypochromic: value falls below the lower limit of the reference interval, red cells have less than average amount of hemoglobin concentration

♥ Hyperchromic: value is above the upper end of the reference interval, red blood cells contain greater than average hemoglobin concentration.

Red Blood Cell Terminology

A variety of terms are used to describe hematologic variations of the red cell. The following terms are used to describe red blood cell morphology.

Abnormal variation in size of the red cell is called **anisocytosis**. The following terms are used to describe **anisocytosis** and are often used to describe variation in size or variation of red blood cell volume.

✓ Normocytic-Red cells are of average size, MCV falls with in the reference interval (Figures 5-1 and 5-2).

✓ Microcytic-Red cells are smaller than average size, MCV is less than the lower limit of the reference interval (Figure 5-3).

✓ Macrocytes-Red cells are larger than average size, MCV is greater than the upper limit of the reference interval.

Variation in the shape of the red cell is called **poikilocytosis**. Abnormally shaped red blood cells are called **poikilocytes** (Figure 5-4). A variety of terms are used to connote specific red blood cell shapes and may be associated with specific disease states.

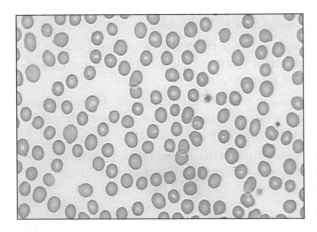

Figure 5-1
Normocytic red blood cells in a cat peripheral blood smear (modified Wright's stain, 100X).

Figure 5-2
Normocytic red blood cells from a dog peripheral blood smear (modified Wright's stain, 100X).

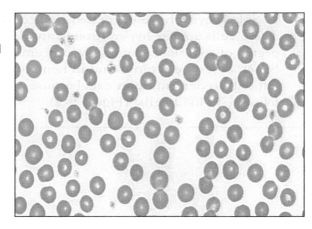

Figure 5-3
Anisocytosis, microcytes, and macrocytes in dog red blood cells peripheral blood smear (modified Wright's stain, 100X).

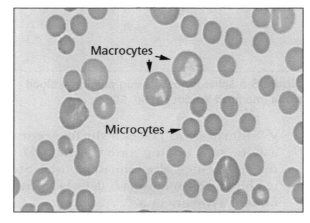

Figure 5-4
Poikilocytosis in dog red blood cell peripheral smear (modified Wright's stain, 100X).

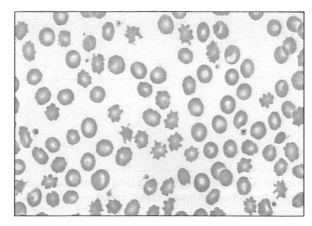

✓ Spherocytes have decreased surface to volume ratio. These cells appear hyperchromic and lack central pallor. The degree of spherical shape may vary among red cells. Spherocytes are often found in hemolytic anemias, but are difficult to determine in cats because of the small size of feline red blood cells. (Figure 5-5).

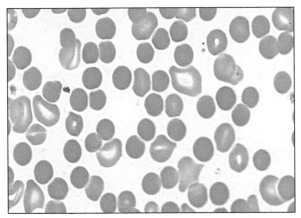

Figure 5-5 Spherocytes in a dog peripheral blood smear (modified Wright's stain, 100X).

✓ Stomatocytes posses a slit-like central pallor surrounded by a dense surrounding zone (Figure 5-6). This gives the cell the appearance of a human mouth. Stomatocytes result from red blood cell membrane defects. These cells may be present in hemolytic anemia.

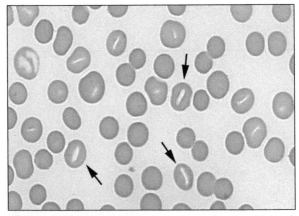

Figure 5-6 Stomatocytes in a dog peripheral blood smear (modified Wright's stain, 100X).

✔ Echinocytes have multiple rounded edge protrusions or spicules, which may be blunt or sharp distributed evenly throughout the red blood cell (Figure 5-7). Echinocytes with blunt spicules are also known as crenated red blood cells. Although these cells are often an in vitro artifact, echinocytes may also occur due to various metabolic disorders.

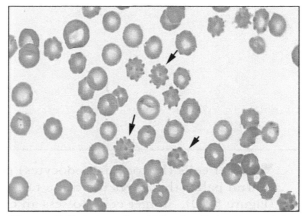

Figure 5-7 Crenated red blood cells in dog peripheral blood smear (modified Wright's stain, 100X).

♥ Burr cells are echinocytes with multiple pointed end spicules (Figure 5-8). Burr cells are produced by a rupture of the cell membrane. They may be seen in renal disease.

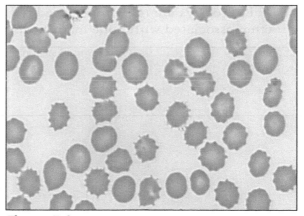

Figure 5-8 Burr cells in dog peripheral blood smear (modified Wright's stain, 100X).

♥ Acanthocytes have multiple irregularly shaped finger-like spicules (Figure 5-9). Acanthocytes are frequently associated with liver disease.

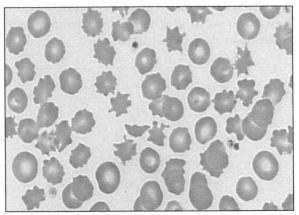

Figure 5-9
Acanthocytes in dog peripheral blood smear (modified Wright's stain, 100X).

♥ Target cells (leptocytes, codocytes) possess a unique central pallor that gives the cell a target-like appearance (Figure 5-10). Target cells possess an excess of cell membrane in relation to the amount of hemoglobin. Target cells are often observed in liver disease.

✓ Ovalocytes or elliptocytes, are oval in shape and possess an oval central pallor (Figure 5-11).

✓ Keratocytes are cells with two horn-like protrusions (Figure 5-12).

♥ Similar cells which contain an arch of membrane between the two projections are known as blister cells.

✓ Dacrocytes are tear drop-shaped red blood cells and are often associated with bone marrow disorders (Figure 5-13).

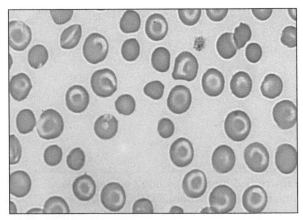

Figure 5-10
Target cells in a dog peripheral blood smear (modified Wright's stain, 100X).

Figure 5-11
Ovalocytes in a cat peripheral blood smear (modified Wright's stain, 100X).

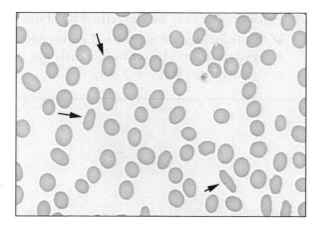

Figure 5-12
Keratocytes in a dog peripheral blood smear (modified Wright's stain, 100X).

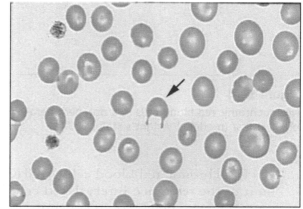

✓ Schistocytes are red blood cell fragments. Schistocytes result from red cell membrane damage during circulation, often a result of microvascular abnormalities. Schistocytes are often seen in disseminated intravascular hemolysis (DIC).

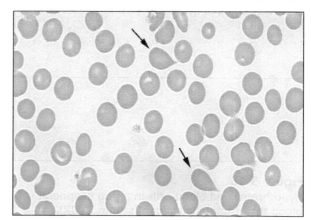

Figure 5-13
Dacrocytes in a dog peripheral blood smear (modified Wright's stain, 100X).

Red blood cells may be described by their hemoglobin content.

✔ Normochromic red blood cells- MCHC falls within the reference interval, red blood cells are of average hemoglobin concentration (Figure 5-14).

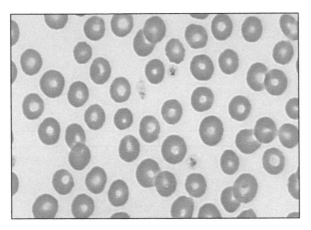

Figure 5-14
Normochromic red blood cells in a dog peripheral blood smear (modified Wright's stain, 100X).

✔ Hypochromic red blood cells-MCHC falls below the lower limit of the reference interval, red cells have less than average amount of hemoglobin concentration (Figure 5-15).

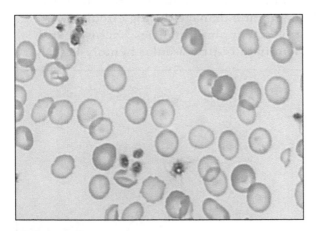

Figure 5-15
Hypochromic red blood cells in a dog peripheral blood smear (modified Wright's stain, 100X).

✔ Hyperchromic red blood cells-MCHC is above the upper end of the reference interval, red blood cells contain greater than average hemoglobin concentration (Figure 5-16). Hyperchromasia is associated with hemolysis and with the presence of spherocyles.

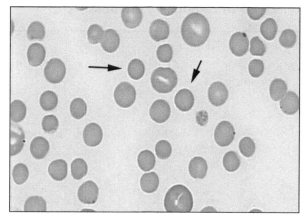

Figure 5-16
Hyperchromic red blood cells in a dog peripheral blood smear (modified Wright's stain, 100X).

✔ Polychromatophilic red blood cells (polychromasia) are larger than mature red blood cells and stain bluish gray (Figure 5-17). These young cells are reticulocytes when stained with New Methlyene Blue.

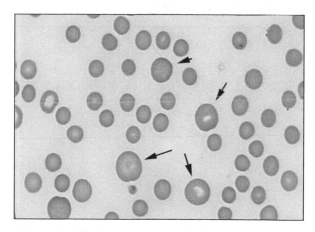

Figure 5-17
Polychromatophilic red blood cells in a dog peripheral blood smear (modified Wright's stain, 100X).

Red Blood Cell Inclusions

♥ Basophilic stippling appears as variably sized blue granules within the red blood cell. In most cases, these granules are residual RNA and represent reticulocytosis. Basophilic stippling may also result from lead poisoning (Figure 5-18). It may also be odserved in responsive anemias.

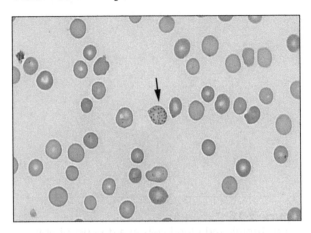

Figure 5-18 Basophilic stippling in a dog peripheral blood smear (modified Wright's stain, 100X).

✔ Howell Jolly Bodies are dark purple red cell inclusions and are approximately 1 μm in diameter. These inclusions are remnant fragments of nuclear chromatin and are often found in responsive anemia patients with splenic disorders, and in splenectomized patients (Figure 5-19).

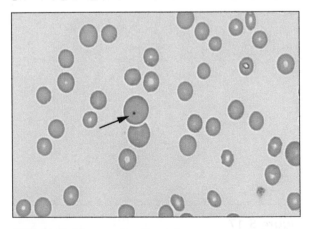

Figure 5-19 Howell Jolly Body in a cat peripheral blood smear (modified Wright's stain, 100X).

✓ Heinz Bodies are not easily identified on Wright's stained blood films, but when stained with New Methylene Blue, appear as pale blue inclusions (Figures 5-20 and 5-21). These inclusions are 1-4 μm in diameter. Heinz bodies are formed in red blood cells when hemoglobin denatures and precipitates. This can be a result of oxidative injury.

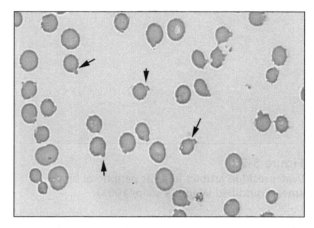

Figure 5-20 Heinz Body in a cat peripheral blood smear (modified Wrights's stain, 100X).

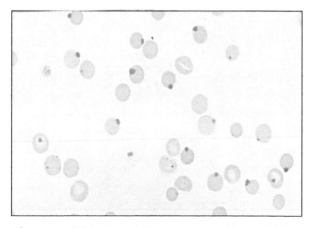

Figure 5-21 Heinz Bodies in a cat peripheral blood smear (New Methelyne Blue stain, 100X).

✓ Water residue appears as refractile inclusions and often vary in size and shape. This artifact is a result of inappropriate staining technique (Figure 5-22).

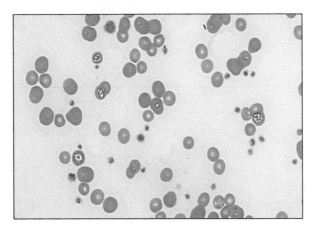

Figure 5-22
Water residue artifact in a cat peripheral blood smear (modified Wright's stain, 100X).

✓ Stain precipitate appears as variably sized purple granules (Figure 5-23). These granules may be concentrated in one area of the smear, or may be distributed throughout the smear. This artifact may be avoided by proper staining techniques.

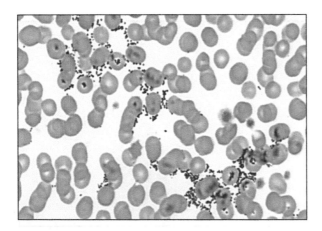

Figure 5-23
Stain precipitate artifact in a dog peripheral blood smear (modified Wright's stain, 100X).

Blood Parasites

✓ Blood parasites may be found in peripheral blood smears (Figures 5-24 and 5-25).

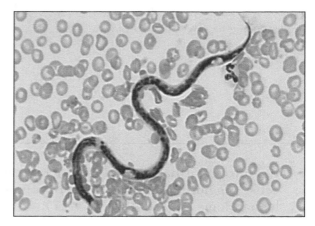

Figure 5-24
Heartworm in a dog peripheral blood smear (modified Wright's stain, 100X).

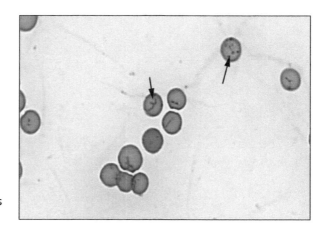

Figure 5-25
Mycoplasma haemofelis in a cat peripheral blood smear (modified Wright's stain, 100X).

Cellular Organization on the Peripheral Blood Smear

✓ Cellular overlap occurs in areas of the peripheral blood smear where red cells, white cells and platelets are not evenly distributed. This artifact may be mistaken for red cell inclusions.

✓ Rouleaux is the "stacked coin" appearance of red cells (Figure 5-26). This description denotes an organized linear array of red cells that is more common in cats. Rouleaux can be an abnormal finding and is associated with inflammatory disease.

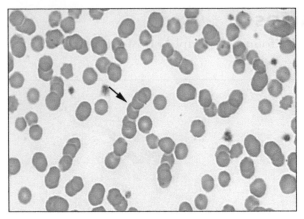

Figure 5-26
Rouleaux in a cat peripheral blood smear (modified Wright's stain, 100X).

✓ Autoagglutination is clumping or aggregates of red blood cells. Agglutination may be seen in immune-mediated hematologic diseases (Figure 5-27).

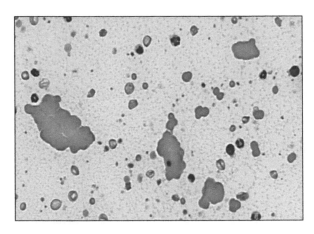

Figure 5-27
Autoagglutination in a cat peripheral blood smear (modified Wright's stain, 50X).

Red Blood Cell Production

Red blood cells are produced in the bone marrow. Presence of immature red cells in the peripheral blood, especially nucleated red cells without commensurate polychromasia, indicates pathology.

✓ Rubriblast-large cell with large, round nucleus, granular chromatin, prominent nucleoli, dark blue cytoplasm (Figure 5-28).

Figure 5-28
Rubriblast in a dog peripheral blood smear (modified Wright's stain, 100X).

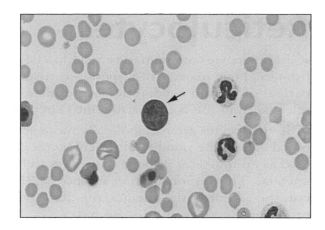

✓ Prorubricyte-large cell, often as large or larger than the rubriblast, round nucleus with ill defined or no nucleoli, coarse chromatin; cytoplasm is predominately blue, but has tinges of red (Figure 5-29).

✓ Rubricyte-smaller than the prorubricyte, round nucleus with no nucleoli; nucleus contains clumps of chromatin and cytoplasm is predomately blue, but has increasing amounts of red.

✓ Metarubricyte-smaller then the rubricyte; nucleus is eccentric, small, and has dense chromatin; cytoplasm is reddish blue.

✓ Polychromatophilic erythrocyte-small cell, no nucleus; cytoplasm is blue to reddish blue depending on maturity.

✓ Mature red blood cell-small cell, stains red, biconcave disc, central pallor.

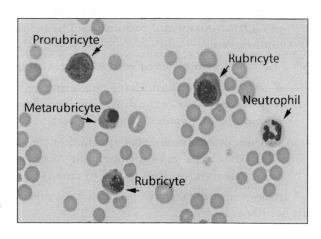

Figure 5-29
Prorubricyte, rubricyte, metarubricyte, and segmented neutrophil in a dog peripheral blood smear (modified Wright's stain, 100X).

Reticulocytes

✓ Reticulocytes are immature red blood cells that are released from the bone marrow in response to tissue hypoxia. During periods of intense need, reticulocytes may be prematurely released from the bone marrow into circulation.

✓ Reticulocytes are metabolically more active than mature red blood cells. The number of reticulocytes in circulation can be used as an indicator of bone marrow activity and its response to anemia. This response varies by species, the type of anemia present, the extent of the anemia, the duration of anemia, and the presence of concurrent disease states.

✓ Reticulocytosis is the hallmark of intensified red blood cell production.

Laboratory Findings

✓ Reticulocytes are anuclear immature red blood cells that contain a characteristic intracellular pattern when stained with supravital stain. Reticulocytes may be quantified by automated or manual methods. Flow cytometry is employed in automated methods. To quantify reticulocytes using the manual method, an anticoagulated blood sample is incubated with supravital stain and a blood smear is prepared. Reticulocytes are counted microscopically.

Microscopic Identification

✓ Residual ribonucleic acid, mitochondria, and organelles of the red blood cell stain dark purple within light blue red blood cells when stained with the supravital stain New Methylene Blue.

♥ When stained with Wright's stain, reticulocytes appear as polychromatophilic red cells. These cells are frequently macrocytic.

✓ There are **two types of reticulocytes: aggregate** and **punctate.**

✓ **Aggregate reticulocytes** are larger cells in size and possess residual nuclear reticulum that appears as a coarse or "lacey" intracellular pattern (Figure 5-30).

✓ **Punctate reticulocytes** are smaller red cells and have residual RNA that appears as intracellular "dots" or "granules." This type of reticulocyte is often found in cats (Figure 5-31).

✓ In dogs and cats, there are small number of reticulocytes present in health.

Figure 5-30
Aggregate reticulocytes in a dog peripheral blood smear (New Methylene Blue stain, 100X).

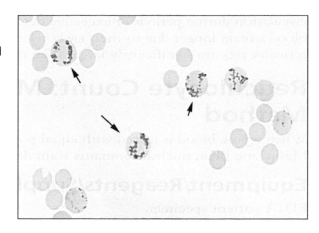

Figure 5-31
Punctate and aggregate reticulocytes in a cat peripheral blood smear (New Methylene Blue stain, 100X).

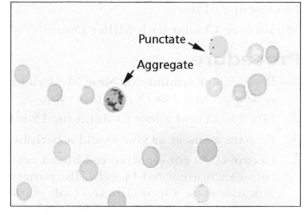

✓ Reticulocyte response is dependent on many factors, including the species, the severity, type and duration of anemia, and concurrent disease.

✓ During regenerative anemia, dogs respond vigorously with aggregate reticulocytosis.

Punctate reticulocytes are present, but are too few to enumerate separately from aggregate reticulocytes.

✓ Both aggregate and punctate reticulocytes are present in the cat. Aggregate reticulocytes mature into punctate reticulocytes within 12 hours of release from the bone marrow. Punctate reticulocytes mature into erythrocytes in approximately 10 days. Most laboratories will either enumerate reticulocytes separately or enumerate aggregate reticulocytes only.

✓ **Shift reticulocytes** are reticulocytes that are released from the bone marrow prematurely. These reticulocytes are released into circulation during periods of excessive demand and persist in the blood stream longer due to their early release. Generally, shift reticulocytes are significantly larger than mature red cells.

Reticulocyte Count: Manual Method

When whole blood is mixed with equal portions of New Methylene Blue, nuclear remnants stain deep blue.

Equipment/Reagents/Supplies

EDTA patient specimen

New Methylene Blue

Microscope Slides

Microscope Ocular with Miller Disc

Procedure

1. Place equal volumes of New Methylene Blue and patient specimen in a 12x75 mm test tube.

2. Mix blood and allow to stand for 15 minutes.

3. Prepare a smear as you would a peripheral blood smear.

4. Count 1000 consecutive red blood cells, differentiating between normal red blood cells, punctate, and aggregate reticulocytes. Optimally red cells should be counted in the monolayer where cells do not overlap.

5. Calculate the two reticulocyte types and report as percentage.

Means of Enumeration

Reticulocytes may be reported as percentage, absolute count, corrected reticulocyte percentage, or reticulocyte production index.

Reticulocyte Percentage

✓ This value is obtained in #5 from the procedure outlined above.

♥ In anemic patients, this method of enumeration often depicts a falsely increased reticulocyte response. This is due to the fact that there are fewer mature red blood cells in circulation and thus appears as a relative increase of reticlocyte response. The presence of shift reticulocytes may also account for an increased reticulocyte percentage.

Absolute Reticulocyte Count

✔ The absolute reticulocyte count is calculated by multiplying the reticulocyte percentage by the red blood cell count.

✔ This method corrects for the relative increase discussed for reticulocyte percentage.

Corrected Reticulocyte Percentage

✔ The Corrected Reticulocyte Percentage is calculated by multiplying the Reticulocyte Percentage by the quotient of the patient's PCV divided by the species specific "normal" PCV.

Reticulocyte Production Index (RPI)

✔ The reticulocyte production index is calculated by dividing the corrected reticulocyte percentage by the reticulocyte maturation time. This corrects for the premature release of shift reticulocytes, which varies with the degree of anemia. For dogs, the reticulocyte maturation time is: PCV 45% = 1 day, PCV 35% = 1.5 days, PCV 25% = 2 days, PCV 15% = 2.5 days.

✔ In dogs, an RPI of ≤ 1 indicates non-regenerative anemia, between 1 and 2 indicates an active and responsive bone marrow, > 2 indicates accelerated erythropoiesis, and ≥ 3 indicates significant regenerative response associated with hemolytic anemia (response to hemolysis or hemorrhage.)

Blood Smear Evaluation Guidelines

1. Using low magnification, scan the entire smear for quality. Poorly stained smears should not be used.

2. Find the counting area. This is the area known as the monolayer (or monolayered area) that has few to no red cells overlapping each other and white cells that are well flattened but not distorted. Red cells may be widely dispersed if the red blood cell count is decreased.

3. Perform a differential white blood cell count.

4. Evaluate neutrophil abnormalities using Table 5-1.

5. Evaluate red blood cell morphology using Table 5-2.

6. Estimate and confirm the platelet count using Table 5-3. Platelet clumps should be reported if present. (Reference intervals vary; these ranges may need to be adjusted accordingly.)

Table 5-1
Neutrophil Abnormalities: Average Number in 100X Field

SEVERITY	NEUTROPHIL ABNORMALITIES	FREQUENCY	
Slight	Cytoplasm foamy. Mild diffuse or focal basophilia. Döhle bodies in cats are considered a slight toxic change.	Few	1-10%
Mild	Cytoplasm foamy to vacuolated. Moderate to marked diffuse or focal basophilia. Döhle bodies.	Moderate	11-50%
Marked	Cytoplasm foamy. Mild diffuse or focal basophilia.	Many	51-100%

Table 5-2
Red Blood Cell Morphology: Average Number in 100X Field

RED CELL MORPHOLOGIC CHARACTERISTIC	SLIGHT	MODERATE	MARKED
Polychromasia: Dog	2-7%	8-14%	>14
Polychromasia: Cat	1-2%	3-8%	>8
Hypochromasia	1-10%	11-50%	>50
Target Cells	1-5%	6-15%	>15
Spherocytosis, Microcytosis, Macrocytosis	1-10%	11-50%	>50
Schistocytes, Acanthocytes, Heinz Bodies, Basophilic Stippling, Other Poikilocytes	1-2%	3-8%	>8

Table 5-3
Platelet Estimate: Average Number in 100X Field

SPECIES	MARKEDLY DECREASED	DECREASED	WITHIN REFERENCE INTERVAL	INCREASED
Dog	<3	4-9	10-25	>26
Cat	<3	4-14	15-40	>41

Section 6
Platelets

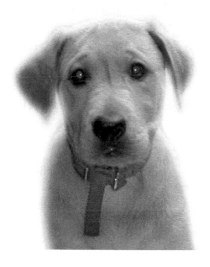

Platelet Structure and Function

Structure

✓ The platelet is discoid in shape and contains no nucleus.

⊙ When Wright's stained, the platelet appears light purple and contains small red-purple granules. The platelet may possess fine thread-like projections (Figures 6-1, 6-2, and 6-3).

✓ The size of the platelet ranges from 5 to 7 μm long and 3 μm wide.

✓ The mean platelet volume of the dog platelet is approximately 8 femtoliters.

✓ The mean platelet volume of the cat platelet is approximately 15 femtoliters.

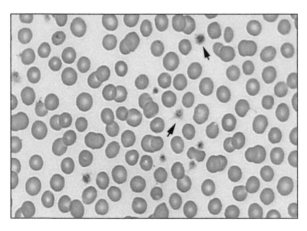

Figure 6-1
Cat platelets in a peripheral blood smear (modified Wright's stain, 100X).

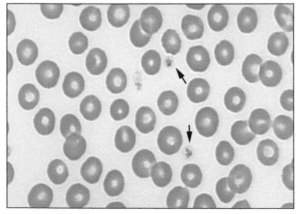

Figure 6-2
Dog platelets in a peripheral blood smear (modified Wright's stain, 100X).

Figure 6-3
Large platelets in dog peripheral blood smear (modified Wright's stain, 100X).

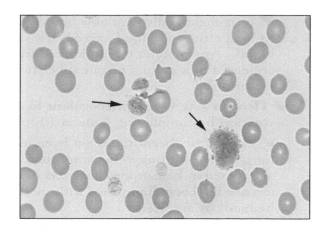

Function

✓ The platelet is a multifunctional cellular element of the blood system. Platelets help maintain vascular integrity, modulate inflammatory response, and promote wound healing after tissue damage.

💣 The most important function of the platelet is its role in hemostasis. Platelets assist in stopping hemorrhage since they are the first cellular element of peripheral blood to react when blood vessels are damaged.

Laboratory Analysis

Specimen Collection

✓ Blood specimens should be collected using routine phlebotomy technique.

✓ Whole blood is necessary for obtaining platelet counts, as platelets are consumed during the clotting process. **EDTA** is the anticoagulant of choice, although **citrate** and **heparin** may be used.

   ✓ **EDTA** acts as an anticoagulant by chelating calcium. Calcium is necessary for the coagulation cascade to proceed; its absence ceases the coagulation process. EDTA is the most commonly used anticoagulant for collection of blood specimens for platelet counts.

   ✓ **Citrate** also acts as an anticoagulant by calcium chelation and is commonly used as the anticoagulant of choice for coagulation studies. In cases of ETDA-dependent platelet agglutination, sodium citrate may be used for obtaining platelet counts.

♥ In commercially available blood tubes, the dilution of sodium citrate to blood exceeds the dilution of EDTA to blood. Any platelet count derived from a blood sample collected in a sodium citrate tube should be increased by a factor of 1.1.

✓ **Heparin** acts as an anticoagulant by inhibiting thrombin formation by complexing with antithrombin III.

✓ Historically heparin has *not* been used as an anticoagulant for platelet counting as heparin interfered with the lysing agent used in hematology analyzers of the 1980s. This interference has been diminished with most currently available hematology analyzers.

✓ Another disadvantage is that Wright's stained blood smears made from heparinzed whole blood may produce an artifact: a light blue background that can interfere with microscopic evaluation of blood cells.

💣 Determine the method of platelet counting before choosing the anticoagulant for blood collection.

Platelet Count Methods

✓ There are three methods of performing platelet counts: **manual, electrical impedance** and **flow cytometry**.

Manual

✓ Platelets are counted microscopically using a hemacytometer.

✓ A well-mixed EDTA anticoagulated blood specimen is diluted 1:100 in 1% ammonium oxalate solution. The Unopette system (Becton-Dickinson, Rutherford, NJ) is available commercially.

✓ A hemacytometer is charged and the unit is left undisturbed for 15 minutes. This allows the platelets to settle.

✓ Platelets appear as round or oval cells microscopically.

✓ Platelets are counted in the entire center square of the hemacytometer. If the total number of platelets counted are less than 100, more small squares are counted until at least 100 platelets have been observed.

✓ The number of platelets per cubic millimeter, is calculated by multiplying the total number of platelets counted by 1000.

Sources of Error

✓ Improper dilution technique

✓ Platelet clumping

Electrical Impedance

✓ Most automated hematology analyzers utilize the **electrical impedance method** to determine platelet counts.

✓ Coulter developed and first marketed the electrical impedance machine in the early 1960s. This method is no longer limited to Coulter instruments and is widely used today.

✓ In automated systems using electrical impedance, anticoagulated whole blood is diluted in an electrolyte solution. The resulting solution of blood cells are routed through a small opening between two electrodes. This opening is known as the aperture. A precise volume of diluted blood is moved through the aperture for a precise time period. As platelets are moved across the aperture, they inhibit the flow of electrical current across that aperture. The detected changes in current are counted as platelets. These changes are accumulated by the instrument and ultimately reported as the platelet count.

Sources of Error

✓ Platelets are sized by amplification of the pulse generated from platelet movement across the aperture. The amplified pulse is compared with internal reference voltage channels. These channels only accept pulses of a certain amplitude; this sorts the pulses into size channels. A histogram is generated from this data which compares cell size to the number of cells present. An algorithm is applied to these data. This sets an upper and lower size limit, or threshold, that is used to discriminate between cell populations.

✓ For most hematology analyzers, the platelet threshold is based on the platelet size of the human species, even if the analyzer has veterinary applications. Cells in the 2-20 femtoliter range are counted as platelets; those counted above 35 femtoliters are counted as red cells. This presents a problem when attempting to obtain platelet counts in species that possess small red cells, as the counting area between platelets and red cells may overlap. This is generally not a problem in red cell counts, as red cell counts are in millions per microliter. However, this may adversely effect the platelet count, as platelet counts are reported in thousands per microliter.

💣 It is therefore imperative to confirm all platelet counts microscopically with a stained peripheral blood smear.

Flow Cytometry

✓ Laser flow cytometry is the newest method of automated platelet counting.

✓ Using flow cytometry, a suspension of anticoagulated whole blood is passed through a laser beam.

✓ All blood cells adsorb and scatter laser light. Each cell type may be classified based on cell size, nuclear components, and cytoplasmic inclusions. Platelets may be counted accordingly.

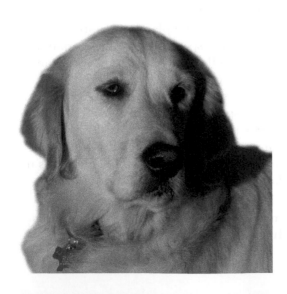

Appendix

Equipment Manufacturers and Suppliers

Bayer Corporation
Elkhart, IN 46515
http://www.bayer.com/en/tk/healthcare.php

Abbott Laboratories
100 Abbott Park Road
Abbott Park, IL 60064-3500
http://www.abbottdiagnostics/com/systems_tests/path.cfm

Idexx
1 Idexx Drive
Westbrook, ME 04092
http://idexx.com

Heska
1613 Prospect Parkway
Fort Collins, CO 80525
http://heska.com

Southeast Vetlab
18131 SW 98th Ct.
Miami, FL 33157
http://www.vetlab.com/

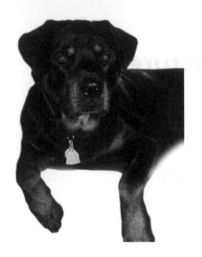

Index

Page numbers followed by an *f* indicate a figure; page numbers followed by a *t* indicate a table.

Blood collection tube, 48

Blood smear, evaluation guidelines for, 99-100

Blood specimen
collection method for, 48
collection of, 78
manual testing procedures for, 49-62
sources of error in, 51
storage and refrigeration of, 48

Blood test
expected values in, 16
false positive and negative readings in, 16
limitations of, 15
methodology of, 15

Bone marrow
dacrocytes in disorders of, 86
red blood cell production in, 94-95

Brightfield microscopy, 21

Bromsulfophthalene, 12

Buffy coat, 51-52

Burr cells, 85

C

Calcium carbonate crystal, 31
chemical confirmation of, 34t

Calcium chelation, 103

Calcium oxalate crystal, 31, 32, 33
chemical confirmation of, 34t

Calcium phosphate, 31

Capillaria plica, 41

Capillary tube
heparinized, 50
macroscopic examination of, 51-52
for microhematocrit method, 52
in micromethod, 50
non-heparinzed, 50

Carbon dioxide, 78

Casts, 27-28
epithelial cell, 29-30
fatty, 29
formation of, 27-28
granular, 28-29
hyaline, 28
red blood cell, 31
reference range for, 45
waxy, 30
white blood cell, 31

Catheterization, 4
bacterial infection with, 40

CBC. See Complete blood count

Cellular degeneration, 31

Cellular organization, on peripheral blood smear, 93-94

Cellular overlap, 93

Centrifugation, 8, 20
of capillary tube, 50
procedure for, 20-21

Centrifuge, 52

Cephalexin, 18

Cephalothin, 18

Chemical analysis, 7-8
procedure for, 8-9

Chemotaxis, 64

Chloride, high concentrations of, 54

Chlorpromazine, 15

Chromatin
fine open, 74
nuclear, fragments of, 90

Citrate, 103

Clot formation, 54

Coagulation factor, plasma concentration of, 53

Cocci, 39

Codocytes, 86

Collection methods, 4
for hematology, 48

Color chart, 7

Color guidelines, 5-6

Color indicator, 7

Complete blood count (CBC), 49

Containers, characteristics and capacity of, 4

Coulter instruments, 79, 105

Cover slip method, 56

Crenated red blood cells, 85

Critoseal, 50, 52

Crystalluria, 31

Crystals
ammonium urate, 36, 37f
amorphous, 32
bilirubin, 36, 37f
calcium carbonate, 36
calcium oxalate, 33
chemical confirmation of, 34-35t
cystine, 38
hippuric acid, 33
leucine, 38
solubility of, 32
triple phosphate, 31, 36, 37f
tyrosine, 38
uric acid, 33
in urine sediment, 31-38

Cystine crystal, 32
chemical confirmation of, 35t
urine pH and, 31

Glomerulonephritis, 31

Glove powder, 42f

Glucose
  in false negative leukocytes test, 18
  high concentrations of, 54
  reference range for in dry chemical
    analysis, 44

Glucose oxidase, 12

Glucose test
  expected values in, 13
  false positive and negatives
    readings in, 13
  limitations of, 12
  methodology of, 12

Glucosuria, 13

Glycoprotein, 11

Granular casts, 28-29

Granules
  basophilic, 60
  eosinophilic, 60
  neutrophilic, 60
  of stain precipitate, 92

Granulocytes, 71

Granulocytic leukocytes, 18

Granulocytic series, 74-76

H

HCT. *See* Hematocrit

Heartwom, 93f

Heinz bodies, 91

Helminthes, eosinophils killing, 67

Hemacytometer, 79, 104

Hematocrit
  definition of, 49
  indirect method of measuring, 51
  procedures for, 49-51
  sources of error in, 51

Hematocrit centrifuge, 55

Hematocrit/packed cell volume, 52-53

Hematology
  specimen collection in, 48
  specimen testing in, 49-62

Hematology analyzer, 105

Heme groups, 78

Hemoglobin, 78
  automated analysis of, 80
  average concentration of, 81-82
  average weight of, 81
  concentration of, 88
  denatured and precipitated, 91
  manual analysis of, 80
  peroxidase activity of, 15

Hemolysis, 53-54

Hemorrhage
  chronic, 54
  platelets in stopping, 103

Hemorrhagic cystitis, 13

Heparin, 104

Heparinzed whole blood, plasma
  from, 53

Hepatic disease, 54

Hippuric acid crystal, 31, 33

Histoplasmosis, 66

Hormones, plasma concentration of, 53

Howell Jolly bodies, 90

Hyaline casts, 28
  with red blood cells, 31

Hyperchromasia, 89

Hyperglycemia, 13

Hypersegmented neutrophils, 72

Hypovolemia, 54

I

Icterus, 53-54

Immune-mediated hematologic disease
  agglutination in, 94
  globulin in, 54

Immunocyte, 73

Immunoglobulin, low production of, 54

Inclusions, red blood cell, 90-92

Indoxyl, 18

Inflammation
  epithelial cells in, 27
  globulin in, 54
  renal, 28
  Rouleaux in, 93

Inflammatory process
  platelets in, 103
  white blood cells in, 71

Ionic concentration indicators, 7

Ionic concentration methodology, 17-18

K

Keratocyte, 86, 87f

Ketone
  in false specific gravity
    elevations, 18
  reference range for in dry chemical
    analysis, 44

Ketones test
  expected values in, 12
  false positive and negative
    reactions in, 12
  limitations of, 12
  methodology of, 11

Kidney, suppurative process in, 31

L

Laboratory analysis
    of platelets, 103-106
    of red blood cells, 79-82
    of reticulocytes, 96

Laser flow cytometry, 106

Leishmaniasis, 66

Leptocyte, 86

Leucine crystal, 35*t*

Leukocyte
    classification of, 60
    in EDTA blood specimens, 48
    reference range for in dry chemical
      analysis, 44
    toxic change in, 71-72

Leukocyte count, abnormal, 51

Leukocyte differential analysis, smear
    preparation for, 57

Leukocytes test
    expected values in, 18
    false positive and negative readings
      in, 18
    limitations of, 18
    methodology of, 18

Lipemia
    cloudy plasma in, 52
    interfering with plasma protein
      reading, 53-54

Lipid degeneration, cellular, 29

Liver disease
    acanthocytes and target cells in, 86
    tyrosine crystalluria and, 31

Lymphocyte, 22
    atypical, 73
    description of, 65
    function of, 65
    in peripheral blood smears, 67*f*
    reactive, 73

M

Macromethod, 50

Macrophage, 66

Manual testing procedures, 49-62

Mass, calcium carbonate crystals in, 36

Mast cells, 73

Matrix mucoprotein
    in cast formation, 27-28
    precipitation of, 28

Mean cell volume (MCV), 51

Mean corpuscular hemoglobin concetra-
    tion (MCHC), 81-82, 88, 89

Mean corpuscular hemoglobin (MCH),
    80-81

Mean corpuscular volume (MCV),
    80-81

Metamyelocyte, 75, 76*f*

Metarubricyte, 95

Methylene Blue stain (New), 60
    of Heinz bodies, 91*f*
    in reticulocyte count, 98
    of reticulocytes, 96, 97*f*

Microbial peroxidase, 16

Microbiocidal action, 64

Microfilaria
    Dirofilaria immitis, 41
    microscopic examination of, 52

Microhematocrit centrifuge, 50-51

Microhematocrit method, 52-53
    equipment, reagents, and supplies
      for, 52
    principle of, 52

Microhematocrit reader, 52

Micromethod, 50
    macroscopic examination of
      capillary tube using, 51-52

Microscopic analysis
    centrifugation in, 20-21
    procedure for, 20-21
    reference ranges for, 44-45
    of reticulocytes, 96-98
    of urine sediment, 21-43
    urine sediment elements found in,
      21-43

Microvascular abnormalities, 87

Mitochondria, 96

Monocyte, 22
    description of, 66
    function of, 66
    in peripheral blood smears, 67*f*

Monohydrate crystals, 32

Mononuclear cell nucleus, 22

Mucoprotein, 27-28

Mucus threads, 38
    reference range for, 45

Mycoplasma haemofelis, 93*f*

Myeloblast, 74

Myelocyte, 74
    in dog peripheral blood stain, 75*f*

Myoglobin, 15

N

Neoplastic transitional epithelial
    cells, 27

Neutrophil, 22-23
    abnormalities of, 100*t*
    band, 70, 71*f*, 75, 76*f*

cat segmented, in peripheral blood smear, 64f
description of, 64
dog segmented, in peripheral blood smear, 65f
function of, 64
hypersegmented, 72
maturation sequence of, 74-76
segmented, 64, 75, 76f

Neutrophilic granule, 71

Neutrophilic leukocyte, 60

Neutrophilic segments, 64, 75, 76f
fusion of, 23

Nitrate
in false negative blood test, 16
reference range for in dry chemical analysis, 44

Nitrate test
expected values in, 17
false positive and negative readings in, 17
limitations in, 17
methodology of, 17

O

Ovalocyte, 86, 87f

Oxidative injury, 91

Oxidizing contaminant, 16

Oxygen transport, 78

P

Packed cell volume (PCV), 49. See also Hematocrit
macromethod of determining, 50
microhematocrit determination of, 52-53
micromethod of determining, 50, 51-52

Parasite
in red blood cells, 93
reference range for, 45
in urine sediment, 41

Parasite ova, 41

Peripheral blood
immature red cells in, 94-95
neutrophils in, 64

Peripheral blood smear, 56-57
cat monocyte in, 67f
cat segmented neutrophil in, 64f
cellular organization on, 93-94
dog lymphocytes in, 65f, 66f
dog monocyte in, 67f
dog segmented neutrophils in, 65f
estimating total WBC and platelet count from, 62
materials for, 57

methods of preparation of, 56-57
procedure for, 57-58
right thickness of, 59f
staining methods for, 59-62
thickness of, 58
thin, 58f
too thick, 59f

pH
in crystal formation, 31
reference range for, 44

pH test
expected values in, 13-14
false changes in, 14
limitations of, 13
methodology of, 13

Phagocytosis
eosinophils in, 67
neutrophils in, 64

Phenazopyridine, 15

Phosphate
amorphous, 31
urine pH and, 31

Plant material artifact, 42f

Plasma
clear, 53
color and clarity of, 52
fibrinogen in, 55-56
microscopic examination of, 52

Plasma protein, 53-54
in complete blood count, 49
decreased values of, 54
equipment, reagents, and supplies for, 54
increased values of, 54
procedure for, 54-55

Platelet
agglutination of, 103
collection of, 103-104
in complete blood count, 49
estimate of, 100t
function of, 103
laboratory analysis of, 103-106
size of, 102
staining of, 60
structure of, 102
volume of, 102

Platelet count
electrical impedance method of, 105
estimating, 62
flow cytometry in, 106
manual method of, 104
sources of error in, 104

Poikilocyte, 82

Poikilocytosis, 82, 83f

Polychromasia, 89

Polychromatophilic erythrocyte, 95

Polyvinylpyrrolidone, 11

S

Salt concentration, 27

Schistocytes, 87

Seal-Ease, 50, 52

Sealing products, 50, 52

Sediment analysis, 8

Semen, in urine, 39

Sodium, high concentrations of, 54

Sodium citrate, 103

Sodium nitroprusside, 11-12

Specific gravity, 7
    in false negative blood test, 16
    in false positive nitrite test, 17
    reference ranges for, 44

Specific gravity test
    expected values in, 18
    false elevations and decreases in, 18
    limitations of, 18
    methodology of, 17

Specimen
    containers for, 4
    processing of, 5
    procurement of, 4

Specimen collection
    of platelets, 103-104
    of red blood cells, 78

Spectrophotometry, 80

Sperm, 39
    reference range for, 45

Spermatozoa, 39

Spherocyte, 84, 89

Splenic disorders, 90

Spun test microhematocrit (PCV)
    capillary tube, 54, 55

Squamous epithelial cells, 25

Stain precipitate artifact, 92

Staining
    methods of, 59-60
    principles of, 60
    troubleshooting problems of, 61-62

Stercobilinogen, 16

Sternheimer-Malbin stain
    (SEDI-STAIN), 21-22

Stomatocyte, 84

Storage, dry reagent strips, 9-10

Sulfhydryl groups, 12

Sulfonamide crystals, 32

T

Tamm-Horsfall mucoprotein, 27-28

Target cell, 86

Tetracycline, 18

Thrombin, inhibited formation of, 104

Total white cell count, 62

Transparency guidelines, 5-6

Transport protein, 53

Triple phosphate crystal, 37f
    chemical confirmation of, 34t

Tubular cells, desquamation of, 29-30

Tubular flow rate, 27

Tubular lumen, red cell aggregation
    in, 31

Tubulointerstitial disorder, 29

Tyrosine crystal, 32
    chemical confirmation of, 35t

Tyrosine crystalluria, 31

U

Unopette system, 79, 80, 104

Urate
    amorphous, 32
    urine pH and, 31

Urea, high concentrations of, 54

Urethra
    bacterial contamination from, 40
    glucosuria in obstruction of, 13

Uric acid, 31

Uric acid crystal, 33

Urinalysis
    definition of, 5-8
    dry chemistry methodologies
        of, 10-18
    dry reagent strip method procedure
        for, 8-10
    reference ranges for, 44-45
    specimen procurement in, 4-5

Urinary tract, transitional epithelial
    cells lining, 25

Urine
    acidified, 11
    chemical properties of, 7-8
    color and transparency of, 5-6
    color reference range of, 44
    density of, 7
    pH of, 13-14
    physical properties of, 44
    specific gravity of, 7
    specific gravity range for, 44
    transparency range of, 44

Urine sediment
    analysis of, 8
    artifacts in, 42-43
    bacteria in, 39-40
    casts in, 27-31
    crystals in, 31-38

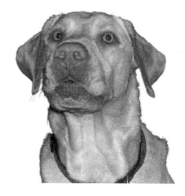

NOTES

NOTES

NOTES